ALLEG HV5138.D78
Drugs and the elderly

3036000000149718

VOID

S0-FFO-449

DATE DUE

FEB 1 1996	
APR 23 '99	

BRODART   Cat. No. 23-221

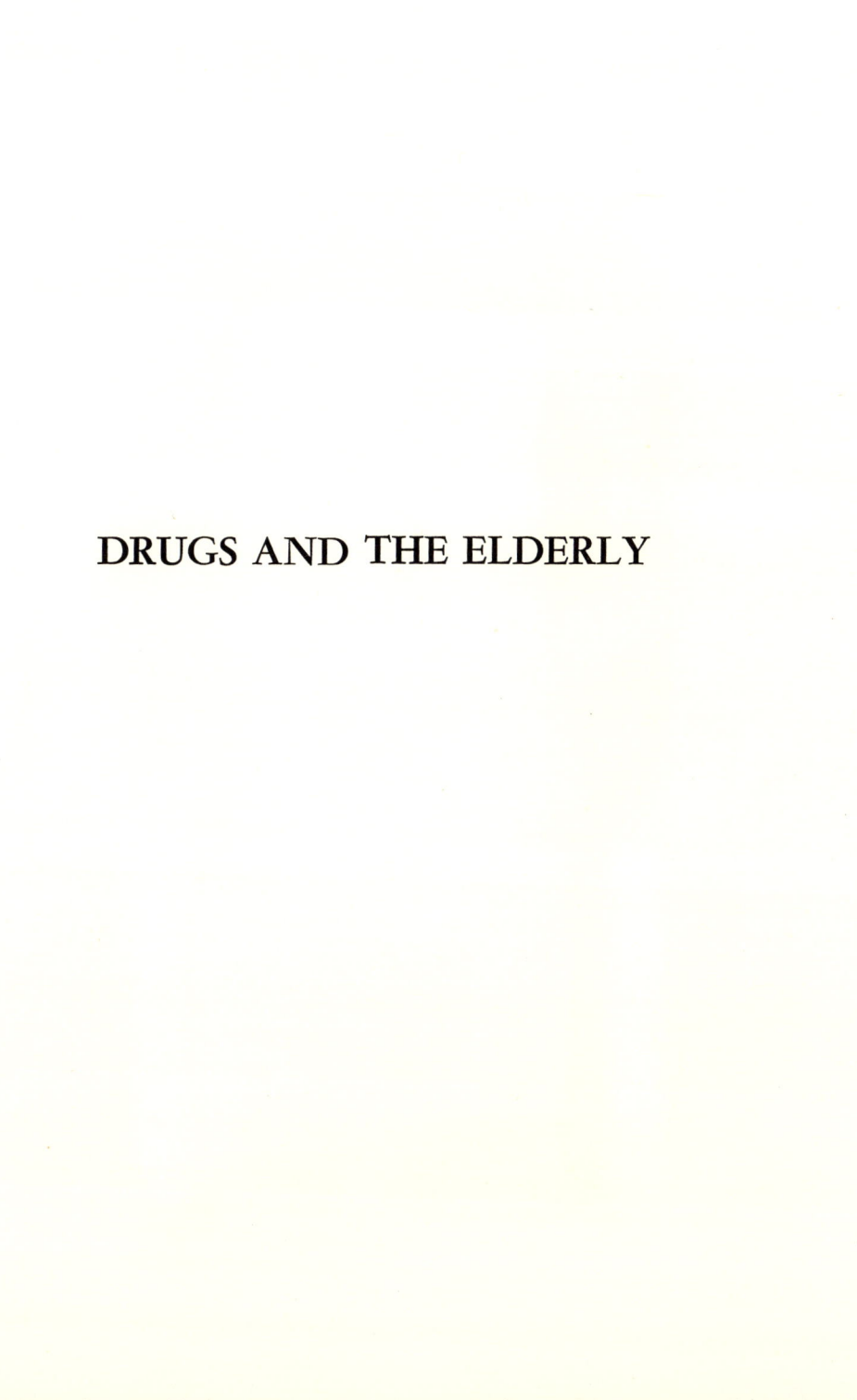

DRUGS AND THE ELDERLY

DRUGS AND THE ELDERLY

Social and Pharmacological Issues

Edited by

DAVID M. PETERSEN, Ph.D.
FRANK J. WHITTINGTON, Ph.D.
BARBARA P. PAYNE, Ph.D.

With a Foreword by

Peter G. Bourne, M.D.

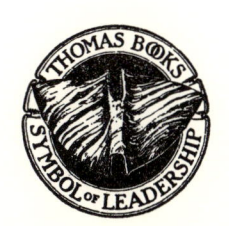

CHARLES C THOMAS • PUBLISHER
Springfield • Illinois • U.S.A.

Published and Distributed Throughout the World by
CHARLES C THOMAS • PUBLISHER
Bannerstone House
301-327 East Lawrence Avenue, Springfield, Illinois, U.S.A.

This book is protected by copyright. No part of it may be reproduced in any manner without written permission from the publisher.

© *1979*, by CHARLES C THOMAS • PUBLISHER
ISBN 0-398-03758-2
Library of Congress Catalog Card Number: 77-17617

With THOMAS BOOKS *careful attention is given to all details of manufacturing and design. It is the Publisher's desire to present books that are satisfactory as to their physical qualities and artistic possibilities and appropriate for their particular use.* THOMAS BOOKS *will be true to those laws of quality that assure a good name and good will.*

Printed in the United States of America
W-2

Library of Congress Cataloging in Publication Data

Main entry under title:

Drugs and the elderly.

Bibliography: p. 221
Includes indexes.
1. Alcohol and the aged—United States—Addresses, essays, lectures.   2. Drugs and the aged—United States—Addresses, essays, lectures.   I. Petersen, David M.
II. Whittington, Frank J.   III. Payne, Barbara.
[DNLM: 1. Drug therapy—In old age. WT100 D794]
HV5138.D78   362.2'92   77-17617

CONTRIBUTORS

PETER G. BOURNE, M.D.: Former positions: Special Assistant to the President, and Director, Office of Drug Abuse Policy; Consultant, Drug Abuse Council; Assistant Director, White House Special Action Office for Drug Abuse Prevention; Special Adviser for Health Affairs to Governor Jimmy Carter; Founder and Director, Atlanta South Central Community Mental Health Center; Consultant, United Nations Division on Narcotic Drugs; Consultant, World Health Division, Geneva. Dr. Bourne is the author of numerous books and articles on mental health, drug abuse, and alcoholism.

CHARLES L. BRAUCHER, Ph.D.: Professor of Pharmacy Care Administration, School of Pharmacy, University of Georgia, Athens, Georgia. He is a member of the Gerontology Faculty (University of Georgia), serving as a member of the Steering Committee and Chairman of the Services Committee. He has been active in pharmaceutical education activities on the national level, having served the American Association of Colleges of Pharmacy as a member of the Board of Directors and as Chairman of the Council of Sections. He is active in mental health activities in Georgia, where he has served as President of the Mental Health Association of Georgia and as a member of the Governor's Advisory Council on Mental Health and Mental Retardation. Dr. Braucher has published numerous articles in pharmacy journals. He received his B.S. degree in Pharmacy from the Philadelphia College of Pharmacy and Science, his M.A. degree in Sociology from the University of Nebraska, and his Ph.D. degree in Pharmacy Administration from Purdue University.

DONALD E. CADWALLADER, Ph.D.: Professor of Pharmacy, School of Pharmacy, University of Georgia, Athens, Georgia. He is a consultant to the Food and Drug Administration and a member of the Scientific Review Panel of the American Pharmaceutical Association Drug Interactions Project. Dr.

Cadwallader is author of a scientific monograph, *Biopharmaceutics and Drug Interactions*. He has contributed chapters to several pharmacy texts and is author of more than fifty scientific and professional articles.

BETSY TODD EPSTEIN, R.N., B.S.N.: Seniors' Health Program, Augustana Hospital, Chicago. Ms. Epstein is a consultant to the Medical College of Pennsylvania and has designed and conducted workshops on drug use among the elderly for consumers and professionals in several states. She is the former health education editor for the *Weekly Review* and has written a series of biweekly health columns for that newspaper. She is co-chairperson of the National Task Force on Drugs and the Elderly and a member of the Health Committee of the Chicago Planning Council on Aging. Ms. Epstein has published several articles and editorials in nursing periodicals and the general press.

RONALD J. GAETANO, B.S., R.Ph.: Executive Director, Broome County Drug Awareness Center, New York. Mr. Gaetano is a consultant to the Medical College of Pennsylvania and has designed and conducted workshops on drug use among the elderly for consumers and professionals in several states. He is President of the National Free Clinic Council; a co-chairperson of the 1977 and 1978 National Drug Abuse Conferences; co-chairperson of the 1977 National Task Force on Drugs and the Elderly; a member of the Drug Advisory Council of the Mental Health Committee of the New York State Assembly; and an educational consultant to the U.S. Civil Service Commission in Department of Health, Education and Welfare Region 2. His publications include a treatise on a program for drug abusers referred by the criminal justice system, a marijuana drug prevention and reading development program for sixth graders, and a book about drug use written for the elderly.

ALBERT W. JOWDY, Ph.D.: Professor and Head, Department of Pharmacy Care Administration, School of Pharmacy, University of Georgia, Athens, Georgia. He has been a member of the Gerontology Faculty since 1968, having served on its council for a number of years. The American Association of Colleges of Pharmacy and the Academy of Pharmaceutical Sciences have been the center of his pharmaceutical education activities. He is a past chairman of the Economic and Administrative Sciences Section and has been elected a Fellow of the Academy. He received his B.S., M.S., and Ph.D. degrees from the University of North Carolina.

GEORGE L. MADDOX, Ph.D.: Professor of Sociology and Director of the Duke University Center for the Study of Aging and Human Development, Durham, North Carolina; a founding member of the Advisory Council of the National Institute on Aging, National Institutes of Health; and President of the Gerontological Society in 1977-1978. Dr. Maddox has written widely on the drinking behavior of adolescents, is coeditor of *Drug Issues in Geropsychiatry,* and is a consulting editor of *The Handbook of Aging and the Social Sciences.*

BARBARA PITTARD PAYNE, Ph.D.: Professor, Department of Sociology, Georgia State University, Atlanta, and Director, Georgia Gerontology Consortium Center. She has held positions with the United Methodist Church as director of adult education, as visiting lecturer and scholar in residence at Emory University and St. Paul's School of Theology, Kansas City, Missouri, and currently is chairman of the section on aging for the Division of Health and Welfare Ministries, Board of Global Ministries of the United Methodist Church. Dr. Payne has coauthored three books, including *Love in the Later Years* (with James A. Peterson), written numerous chapters and articles, and is a contributing editor of *Religious Research Review* and a consulting editor for several publishers. Her current research is a longitudinal study of the older volunteer. Dr. Payne received her master's and doctorate degrees from Emory University, Atlanta, Georgia.

DAVID M. PETERSEN, Ph.D.: Associate Professor, Department of Sociology, Georgia State University, Atlanta, Georgia. He previously taught at the University of South Florida, Ohio State University, and the University of Miami School of Medicine (Division of Addiction Sciences). He is a frequent contributor to the professional literature on the administration of justice, drug addiction, and the sociology of corrections. His most recent book is *Prison Organization and Inmate Subcultures* (with C. W.

Thomas) and is currently working on two additional manuscripts: *The Prison: Socialization in a Coercive Setting* and *The Correctional System: An Introduction* (both with C. W. Thomas).

CHARLES W. THOMAS, Ph.D.: Associate Professor, Department of Sociology, Bowling Green State University, Bowling Green, Ohio. He received his B.S. from McMurry College and his M.A. and Ph.D. degrees from the University of Kentucky. Prior to assuming his present position, he was the Research Director of the Metropolitan Criminal Justice Center at the College of William and Mary and, prior to that, an Assistant Professor with the Department of Sociology at Virginia Commonwealth University. He has contributed numerous articles to a variety of journals in the field of criminology, criminal law, and sociology. His most recent work, coauthored with David M. Petersen, is *Prison Organization and Inmate Subcultures*.

DORIS LANG THOMAS, B.S., M.S.C.: Director, Pharmaceutical Services, Isabella Geriatric Center, New York, New York. Formerly: Chief Pharmacist, Bronx Eye & Ear Infirmary; Owner, Retail Pharmacy; Coordinator, Pilot Projects, American Home Products at Rutgers University; Research Chemist, Signal Corps, U.S. Army, Fort Monmouth, New Jersey; Instructor, Hospital Pharmacy, College of Pharmacy, Columbia University; Consultant to long-term care facilities on pharmaceutical policies and procedures. Mrs. Thomas has done pioneer work in the field of sociopharmaceutics in relationship to resident populations in long-term care facilities and has written several articles on this subject.

JAMES A. THORSON, Ed.D.: Coordinator of Academic Affairs, Gerontology Program, University of Nebraska at Omaha. Formerly: Program Specialist in Gerontology, Georgia Center for Continuing Education, and Assistant Professor of Adult Education, University of Georgia. Dr. Thorson has been chairman of the advisory council on aging for the state of Georgia and is Past-President of the Georgia Gerontology Society. Dr. Thorson is also a Fellow of the Gerontological Society. He has written numerous articles on attitudes toward aging and death and dying and is currently editing a book entitled *Spiritual Well-Being of the Aged* for Charles C Thomas, Publisher.

JUDY R. J. THORSON, R.N., M.Ed.: Consultant in allied health training and nursing. Ms. Thorson specializes in patient education and in the training of paraprofessionals in the health field and has had a variety of professional experiences in the field of nursing, from obstetrics to geriatrics. She received the B.S. and M.Ed. degrees in Health Occupations Education from the University of Georgia and has taught nurse assistants and practical nurses in several vocational-technical institutes.

FLYNN WARREN, M.S.: Clinical Coordinator for Pharmacy Programs, Medical College of Georgia, Augusta, Georgia. Currently Mr. Warren is on leave from the university and serving as Drug Information Pharmacist at the King Faisal Specialist Hospital and Research Centre, Riyadh, Saudi Arabia. Formerly, Instructor in Clinical Pharmacy, School of Pharmacy, University of Georgia, Athens, Georgia. He is a member of various professional, honorary, and scientific organizations and serves on the scientific panels of the American Pharmaceutical Association's drug interactions review program. He has published articles in both professional and scientific journals and has appeared on many seminar faculties. Mr. Warren received his B.S. in Pharmacy from the University of South Carolina and his M.S. in Hospital Pharmacy from the University of Georgia where he is currently completing the requirements for his Ph.D.

FRANK J. WHITTINGTON, Ph.D.: Assistant Professor and Associate Director of Graduate Studies in Aging, Department of Sociology, Georgia State University, Atlanta, Georgia. Dr. Whittington received his doctoral degree from Duke University, where he was a Research Training Program Fellow in the Center for the Study of Aging and Human Development. He has served in several capacities in professional societies, including that of President of the Georgia Gerontology Society. His publications include articles and chapters on the relative socioeconomic status of the aged, mental health care in nursing homes, older women, and drug use among the elderly. He is coauthor with his wife, Susan E. Whittington, of *Georgia's Older Popula-*

tion: A Data Book on Aging. Dr. Whittington's current research is an epidemiological and attitudinal investigation of drug use among the noninstitutionalized elderly.

WILLIAM F. WIELAND, M.D.: Director of Education and Training, Ridgeview Institute, Smyrna, Georgia. Also, Assistant Professor of Clinical Psychiatry, Emory University Medical School, Atlanta, Georgia. Formerly: Medical Director of Georgia Mental Health Institute; Director of Drug Abuse Services, Georgia Department of Human Resources; Director of Division of Addictive Diseases, Department of Public Health, City of Philadelphia, Pennsylvania; Director of Narcotic Addict Rehabilitation Program, Philadelphia, Pennsylvania. His clinical research and publications are primarily in the area of addictive disorders.

RONALD J. ZIANCE, Ph.D.: Assistant Professor of Pharmacology, University of Georgia School of Pharmacy, Athens, Georgia. Dr. Ziance received his B.S. in Pharmacy and his Ph.D. in Pharmacology from the University of Pittsburgh and also served as a Postdoctoral Fellow in Pharmacology at the University of Colorado Medical Center. He has published several research papers dealing with the effects of amphetamine and related drugs on neurotransmitter function in brain tissue.

SHELDON ZIMBERG, M.D.: Director of Psychiatry, Hospital for Joint Diseases and Medical Center, and Associate Professor of Psychiatry, Mount Sinai School of Medicine, New York City. Formerly, Deputy Director, Rockland County Community Mental Health Center, and Chief, Community Psychiatry, Harlem Hospital Center. He is a Diplomate of the American Board of Psychiatry and Neurology (Psychiatry) and Certified Mental Hospital Administrator; Associate Examiner, American Psychiatric Association Committee on Certification in Administrative Psychiatry; Fellow, American Psychiatric Association; Chairman, Committee on Alcoholism and Drug Abuse of the New York County District Branch of the American Psychiatric Association; Fellow, American Public Health Association; Fellow, New York Academy of Medicine; Chairman, Committee on Treatment of Alcoholism of the New York State Alcoholism Planning Task

Force; Chairman, Committee on Alcoholism Inpatient Detoxification Screening Criteria, New York County Health Services Review Organization. Dr. Zimberg is the author of a number of publications on community mental health, geriatric psychiatry, and alcoholism. He is the senior editor of a forthcoming book entitled *Psychotherapy of Alcoholism: Theory and Techniques*.

FOREWORD

Everyone knows about drugs and youth. In the last decade we have been inundated with reports relating to marijuana, LSD, heroin, and the youth culture. It would not be possible to remain unaware that the drug problem is one of the major issues of our time. Yet our view of drug use as predominantly a youth phenomenon is misleading. In the population as a whole, 26 percent of all Americans use some kind of psychoactive drug on a regular basis (at least three times a month), and this excludes alcohol, marijuana, and tobacco. Most of the 50 million people who consume these drugs do so under medical guidance and have some degree of legitimate need for them.

Although doctors prescribe most of these drugs, a significant percentage are not consumed by those for whom they were prescribed, or they are taken in different amounts or for different indications. The housewife who takes diet pills for energy and to relieve depression, the athlete who takes drugs to enhance his performance, or the socially anxious person who borrows pills from a friend to be more comfortable in a social setting, all are to some extent abusing drugs. While we associate the consumption of drugs with youth, the fact is that older people consume disproportionately more of all kinds of drugs than the rest of the population. In addition, this disproportionate consumption is continuing to increase. Comprising only one tenth of the population, those sixty-five and older receive one quarter of all prescriptions written, up from one-fifth in 1965.

What are the reasons for this? First, because of the aging process and increasing physical illness with age, older people, more than any other age-group, are exposed to and consume more drugs than they legitimately need. Moreover, the incidence of psychiatric disorders increases with age. For example, there is a decade-by-decade rise in depression, including the peaking of suicide among men in their eighties. Twenty-five percent of all suicides occur in persons over sixty-five years of age. While the abuse of drugs does not automatically correlate with psychiatric illness, there is a strong tendency at all age-levels for the chronically depressed to turn to drugs (including alcohol) as a way to numb their psychic suffering and to escape from a painful environment with which they cannot deal. There is substantial evidence that barbiturates and tranquilizers are heavily resorted to by older people to cope with depression and are the single most common method of committing suicide. While we do not usually think about suicide as drug abuse in the usual sense, it is one of the most important consequences of having large quantities of drugs on hand.

Not only do older people take a disproportionate percentage of manufactured drugs, they are also more physically susceptible to their effects than younger people. They are less capable of metabolizing most drugs and more susceptible to direct, side, and interactional effects of drugs. Nearly one fifth of the patients entering the geriatric service of one general hospital displayed disorders directly attributable to the effects of prescribed drugs. Most often this is due to a failure to recognize that many older people require smaller quantities of most drugs and hence are prescribed amounts in excess of their needs.

Physicians too often play a significant role in the drug problems of older people. Many are unaware of the sensitivity of older people to powerful drugs. Also with addictive drugs they frequently adopt the attitude that it is all right for an older person to become addicted if it will relieve some discomfort. While the intentions may be good, the problems involved in being addicted can be just as distressing for an older person as for an addict on the street. There may be some legitimacy in prescribing an addictive drug when the older patient is in the terminal stages of an illness, but even then, this course of therapy should be approached with caution. One California physician was quoted as saying when told that an elderly woman was addicted to Percodan®, "She's an old lady, let her enjoy it." This unfortunate attitude implies that drug abuse is a moral issue and that if you are old you have somehow earned the right to sin and pleasure. This is not to say, however, that a person in the terminal stages of an illness should be denied whatever drugs would make him comfortable.

Of greater concern is the role of physicians in overprescribing for nursing home residents. Too often medication is provided not particularly for the benefit of the patient but as a deliberate effort to keep patients subdued so that they create a minimum of disturbance for the staff. Drugs then have become a tool for administrative efficiency. This is unfortunately true not only in nursing homes but also for old people in general who are often provided drugs as an overly simplistic solution to their problems rather than being offered better general services for dealing with the varied problems of aging.

One drug that should certainly not be overlooked when we consider drug use in the aging is alcohol. More abused than all other drugs put together, alcohol is clearly identified as the drug of older generations and is certainly the cause of the greatest social and individual cost. Recently a study was made of elderly arrests in San Francisco, a city where 18 percent of the population is sixty years or older. In this age-group 80 percent of the 2,200 arrests studied were for drunkenness, and an additional 4 percent were for traffic offenses involving alcohol. We all have seen the homeless alcoholic men in the skid row of every city in the country, which should in itself convince us of the seriousness of this problem in the older members of our society.

Too often the use of alcohol is not the result of emotional illness or psychological stress but merely of increased leisure time, boredom, and a lack of challenging activities. Loneliness is a major problem for many people in our society, not merely the aged, but for this group it is probably the most widespread. Combined with chronic debilitation and, in many instances, pain, alcohol offers a pleasant, available, and relatively cheap escape. Of particular significance is the effect of combining drugs with heavy alcohol consumption, which in the elderly can have disastrous results.

Perhaps the biggest problem in attempting to deal with the issue of drug use in the elderly is the almost total lack of awareness by the general population that it exists. Lacking the glamour of LSD and marijuana use by young people, the chronic use of drugs by the aging does not arouse the same emotional reaction. Even among workers in the drug field this is an area that has consistently had a low priority and has consistently been neglected.

Clearly, a top priority must be dissemination of information and a concerted effort to raise the awareness of the general public and those in the helping professions to the problem of drug abuse in the elderly. Having once commanded public attention, it then becomes possible to institute a variety of other steps in dealing with the problem. Much of the problem stems merely from ignorance on the part of physicians and other health professionals. They generally receive little training in gerontology, particularly as it relates to drugs. Pharmacists and physicians need not only to be alerted to the problem but also to be given a deeper understanding of how they can effectively deal with it. In addition, not only do professionals need education, but so also do elderly people themselves. Many older people consume large quantities of drugs completely unaware of the potential hazards, or they unknowingly badger physicians into overprescribing for them drugs which they really do not need. Education for the consumer needs to be an essential ingredient of our overall effort.

We do not know very much about drug abuse in the elderly. Almost all research has been conducted on the young abuser, and we know almost nothing about the older person who turns to drugs and what the natural history of that drug use will be. We need an increased focus in this area so that we can really fully understand the special aspects of this problem in the aging. It is only very recently that there has begun to be any interest in this field. A number of conferences have been held and several publications produced. This volume represents, however, the first effort to provide a comprehensive overview of the field of drug abuse in the elderly.

Above all we need to realize that drug problems cannot be separated from other problems. They are only symptoms of a gamut of other ills, including boredom, loneliness, a sense of rejection and uselessness, and a lack of alternative, fulfilling, and challenging activity. It is only by dealing with all the emotional needs of the aging that we can effectively eliminate the tendency to turn to drugs and alcohol as an elusive and ephemeral solution to the social, psychological, and physical stresses brought by age.

PETER G. BOURNE

PREFACE

THIS VOLUME IS AN outgrowth of a conference on Drugs and the Elderly held at Georgia State University in February, 1975. This conference was attended by professionals working in aging, drug abuse, mental health, and related disciplines, as well as by a large group of older people from the community.

Prior to the conference, none of the editors had been involved in either research or practice in the area of drug use among the elderly. However, much of the senior editor's professional activities had been centered in the area of drug addiction and drug abuse, whereas the other editors were social gerontologists concerned, respectively, with the medical and community behavior of the aged. The conference developed, then, from our mutual recognition of a topic deserving of attention, although, admittedly, we approached the conference only vaguely perceiving the import or dimensions of the problem. Consequently, experts with a wide range of backgrounds, including medicine, psychiatry, pharmacology, pharmacy, sociology, social work, the ministry, and nursing home administration, were assembled to delineate the nature and extent of drug problems among the elderly. During the three days of the conference it became clear that, while quite a lot was known about the effects of the aging process on pharmacological efficacy and safety, very little of this information had been made readily available to those who needed it. In addition, there appeared to be a great lack of knowledge about both patterns and causes of elderly drug misuse that would be useful to the gerontologist, the geriatric specialist, and the community professional. With the needs of these diverse groups in mind, we decided that a practically oriented book on drugs and the elderly was needed and invited the conference participants to contribute to such a volume. In addition, several persons not at the conference were subsequently invited to prepare chapters addressing important issues which had been revealed but not specifically dealt with in the conference. This book, then, is aimed primarily at the professional practitioner, but the academician will also find it of considerable value for undergraduate and graduate courses in both gerontology and drug abuse.

The book is organized into three major topic areas. Section I presents an overview and several perspectives on the problem. Specifically, the major issues surrounding older people's use of drugs are discussed, and the available literature on drug and alcohol use and misuse is surveyed to provide the reader with a summary of the major research findings in this area. Section II is devoted to the subjects of pharmacology and pharmacy as they relate to the elderly and includes chapters on drug side effects, drug interactions, the problems of self-medication, and the practice of community and institutional pharmacy. In Section III, we address clinical and community responses to elderly drug use. Topics include the appropriate responsibility of health care professionals, including physicians and nurses, strategies for educating the elderly drug user and for preventing drug misuse among community elderly, and, finally, social policy concerns and suggestions. A selected bibliography on drug use and misuse among the elderly is included at the end of the volume to facilitate further investigation by the reader.

D.M.P.
F.J.W.
B.P.P.

ACKNOWLEDGMENTS

W E ARE INDEBTED to several people and organizations for their assistance in the preparation of this book. We would first like to acknowledge the Urban Life Center of Georgia State University and the National Institute on Drug Abuse for their financial support of the conference which precipitated this work. We also owe a great debt of appreciation to the contributors to this volume for their hard work and dedication. Finally, we want to thank Jim Wilson, Cheryl Sisk, Carol Brown, and Marie Langley for the many hours they spent in typing the final draft of the manuscript.

D.M.P.
F.J.W.
B.P.P.

CONTENTS

	Page
Contributors	v
Foreword	xiii
Preface	xix
Acknowledgments	xxi

SECTION I.
PERSPECTIVES ON ELDERLY DRUG USE

Chapter
1. DRUGS, PHYSICIANS, AND PATIENTS 5
   George L. Maddox
2. DRUGS AND THE ELDERLY 14
   Frank J. Whittington and David M. Petersen
3. ALCOHOL AND THE ELDERLY 28
   Sheldon Zimberg
4. ACUTE DRUG REACTIONS AMONG THE ELDERLY 41
   David M. Petersen and Charles W. Thomas

SECTION II.
PHARMACOLOGY, PHARMACY, AND THE ELDERLY PATIENT

5. SIDE EFFECTS OF DRUGS IN THE ELDERLY 53
   Ronald J. Ziance
6. DRUG INTERACTIONS IN THE ELDERLY 80
   Donald E. Cadwallader
7. PHARMACEUTICAL SERVICES FOR THE
   ELDERLY PATIENT 94
   Albert W. Jowdy and Charles L. Braucher
8. SELF-MEDICATION PROBLEMS AMONG THE ELDERLY..105
   Flynn Warren
9. CLINICAL AND ADMINISTRATIVE ASPECTS OF
   DRUG MISUSE IN NURSING HOMES 126
   Doris Lang Thomas

Chapter	Page

SECTION III.
CLINICAL AND COMMUNITY RESPONSE TO ELDERLY DRUG USE

10. THE PHYSICIAN'S ROLE IN THE ADMINISTRATION OF PSYCHOTROPIC DRUGS TO THE ELDERLY PATIENT 141
    William F. Wieland
11. NURSING RESPONSIBILITIES IN THE ADMINISTRATION OF DRUGS TO OLDER PATIENTS 151
    James A. Thorson and Judy R. J. Thorson
12. STRATEGIES AND TECHNIQUES FOR DRUG EDUCATION AMONG THE ELDERLY 163
    Ronald J. Gaetano and Betsy Todd Epstein
13. COMMUNITY RESPONSIBILITY FOR DRUG USE BY THE ELDERLY 178
    Barbara P. Payne
14. DRUGS, AGING, AND SOCIAL POLICY 190
    Frank J. Whittington

Selected Bibliography 221
Name Index 235
Subject Index 243

DRUGS AND THE ELDERLY

Section I

PERSPECTIVES ON ELDERLY DRUG USE

Chapter 1

DRUGS, PHYSICIANS, AND PATIENTS*
George L. Maddox, Ph.D.

Early in my career, my research and publications concentrated on the drinking behavior of young people. In the 1950s the drug of interest to professionals was alcohol, because this was the drug of choice among youth as well as among adults that demonstrably had great potential for abuse. Interest in and concern about *substance* abuse as distinct from alcohol or drug abuse was still a decade away. Over the years, my research interests moved increasingly toward the other boundary of adulthood—late life—but, for a number of reasons, my earliest interest in substance abuse (or alcohol or drug abuse) was not maintained. The evidence concerning drinking behavior over the life course seemed to indicate a decrease in the probability of use over time, on one hand, and, on the other, sustained high levels of use in the middle years appeared to increase the risk of death. My disinterest in the use of the particular drug, alcohol, seemed warranted.

To my surprise, in recent years, colleagues who know of my interest in drinking behavior *and* late life have asked me about substance abuse in late life. My inquirers get little help from me. The evidence that substance abuse by older people is a widespread and substantial problem that could be predicted by knowledge of developmental processes in late life is, in my estimation, very weak. This conclusion may not be warranted. However, even if convincing evidence of substance abuse *by* older persons were mobilized, this strikes me as trivial in comparison with another issue of substance abuse which involves older persons,

---
* A portion of this chapter appeared in W. E. Fann and G. L. Maddox (Eds.): *Drug Issues in Geropsychiatry*, 1974. Courtesy of The Williams & Wilkins Co., Baltimore, Maryland.

namely, the abuse *of* older persons by health professionals who use prescription drugs frequently without adequate information and surveillance.

The Duke University Center for the Study of Aging and Human Development, Durham, North Carolina, has been increasingly interested in "drugs and older people" as the magnitude of the problem has become clear. In response, national conferences were convened at the Center to address basic scientific issues in psychopharmacology and aging[2] and the translation of scientific knowledge into practice.[3] These conferences and the related publications highlighted some issues but certainly did not solve them. In January, 1976, the *New York Times* published a series of five articles on what they labeled "incompetent doctors." The third article of that series carried the front page headline "Thousands a Year Killed by Faulty Prescriptions" and began, "Every year perhaps 30,000 Americans accept the drugs their doctors prescribe for them and die as a direct result. Perhaps 10 times as many patients suffer life-threatening and permanent side effects, such as kidney failure, mental depression, internal bleeding, and loss of hearing or vision. These figures are among the conservative to be found in studies of the prescription drug problem by the medical profession itself. . . ."[9]

Older persons are especially likely to be involved with faulty prescriptions as a drug problem, since they are at high risk of multiple illnesses, the management of which is likely to include prescription drugs. Older persons who occupy nearly all of the over one million nursing home beds in the United States are the most vulnerable of all. The Special Committee on Aging of the United States Senate, in a series entitled *Nursing Home Care in the United States: The Failure in Public Policy,* prepared a background paper on drug abuse in nursing homes.[11] The abuse the report discusses is not substance abuse *by* nursing home residents but the abuse *of* residents. The report indicates, "The average nursing home patient takes from four to seven different drugs a day (many taken twice or three times a day). . . Not surprisingly, 20 to 40 percent of nursing home drugs are administered in error. . . . Other serious consequences include: theft and misuse of nursing home drugs; some disturbing evidence of drug addiction; and lack of adequate controls in the regulation of drug experimentation."[11]

The reports from 1975 and 1976 are only the most current illustrations of a substantial drug problem that involves older people. This urgent problem is iatrogenic (caused by those who presumably intend to help). The problem was quite apparent in 1974 when I wrote the opening chapter for the second conference on drugs and older persons at the Duke Center. Nothing has changed since then except, perhaps, increased public awareness. My analysis, then, is repeated in the paragraphs which follow.

* * *

We live in a society which desperately wants to believe that better living can be achieved through chemistry. Informed individuals are now less confident than they once were that their faith is well placed, but the will to believe is still there. Although reliable comparative evidence is limited, Americans have earned a reputation for consuming large quantities of a variety of drugs; some are prescribed, some are not. Members of the younger generation have inherited a culture that generally accepts drugs so casually that we now have a new category of drugs—the recreational ones. When adults remonstrate with the young about the dangers of drugs, the young are quick to point out who has set a national example of excessive drug use. Physicians sometimes wonder aloud about the questionable example they themselves set as tutors of public understanding and taste regarding drugs.[6]

My professional experience with drugs has been primarily with mankind's most ancient, widely used, and frequently abused drug, beverage alcohol. Over the past two decades, my observation of attitudes and behavior related to alcohol has left few illusions about the capacity of either laymen or professionals to do much straight thinking about that drug. Alcohol use is surrounded by venerable myths and a great deal of magic; an essential pragmatism in the use of alcohol underlies our willingness to assume considerable personal risk in the hope that we and the world we perceive can be transformed chemically into something better than they appear to be. My observations about our premier recreational drug proved to be more relevant than one might have expected in understanding my initial year at Duke University Medical Center thirteen years ago.

As a Russell Sage postdoctoral fellow in medical sociology, my objective was to become acquainted with what the Foundation euphemistically called the "culture of a medical school." My point of entry was the Medical Outpatient Clinic at Duke, and it was my good fortune to work with Dr. Morton Bogdonoff, who quickly established himself with me, as well as with his medical students, as a very perceptive clinician and as a physician with a keen interest in clinical research. To begin, Bogdonoff encouraged me simply to sit in the back room—the "pill closet" it was called—and observe the interaction between students who were on their first clinical rotation and their tutors. In spite of the essential seriousness and good sense of these encounters, much of what transpired was the stuff that inspired the successful screen play, $M^*A^*S^*H$. I often wished I had the skill to capture the essence of the humor that pervades the serious business of treating sick people. I remember specifically my curiosity about the way doctors talked about the drugs they handled with great casualness. A typical conversation went like this:

Student: My patient has problem X. In my treatment I plan to use drug Y. That OK?

Tutor: Sure, patients love the blue and pink pills. There are not many specific drugs, you know. The trick is to be sure you do no harm. You ought to check the desk reference for side effects. That's a good practice.

Student: Patients really like the blue and pink ones?

Tutor: Sure do. But watch out for brown ones. The point to keep in mind is that a pill is an extension of you; it's a part of you the patient takes with him. When he says he doesn't like a pill, he's probably talking about you.

The student then left for a quick glance at the desk reference on drug effects.

Such conversations made an impression on me at the time. Were drugs as nonspecific as they appeared to be? Was there as much uncertainty as there appeared to be? My experience over the past decade has increased my awareness that pharmacological management is indeed a high-risk enterprise practiced under conditions of considerable uncertainty. Louis Goodman, in what he calls an exercise in dissection regarding the efficacy of drugs, lists forty-eight variables which probably affect the outcome when physicians, patients, and drugs meet.[4] Twenty of these factors refer to the drug (dosage, absorption, interaction), nine factors refer to the patient (age, weight, metabolism), and nine factors refer to the physician (diagnostic skill, experience with drugs, milieu influences). The scientific mind boggles at the prospect of a research design that could manage adequately even a fraction of the variables mentioned. And perhaps we can appreciate today why in the Homeric epics *pharmakon* meant charm, the effect of which depended mainly on the favor of deity, proper ceremonial observance, and the intent of the person who used the charm. One can only smile sympathetically when reading T. S. Eimerl's estimation of his therapeutic intent, i.e. his certainty about outcome, involving drugs used with his patients over a period of four weeks.[1] Of the 580 cases recorded, 8 percent of drugs prescribed were listed as "specific"; 15 percent, "probable"; 26 percent, "possible"; 21 percent, "hopeful"; and 30 percent, "placebo." We would have been further instructed if Eimerl had included a category "considered medication but was too uncertain to prescribe," although this may be included in the placebo category.

Given the high incidence of drug prescription by physicians and laymen in this country and the uncertainty of knowledge about drug effects on particular individuals, we are probably fortunate that toxic reactions and accidents are not more common than they are. But adverse reactions are common enough. In the past two decades, studies of adverse outcomes ("problems of medical progress" is the euphemism) indicate that a 5 percent incidence of adverse outcomes in a university teaching hospital is not unusual. And in the recent Health, Education and Welfare report by the Commission on Medical Malpractice, an estimated 8 percent of medical and surgical cases result in presumably avoidable injury to the patient.[10] Because many malpractice suits stem from errors in medication by both physicians and nurses, the Commission recommended a "major upgrading in skills," with particular attention paid to courses in clinical pharmacology, which should be required at all levels of training and as a part of continuing education. "It is all very well," writes Joseph Garland, "to expect the practicing physician to make judgements on the uses and toxic side effects of one new product after another, but a trained clinical pharmacologist can hardly keep up with the field and the average physician needs help beyond the smattering of pharmacology he acquired in medical school."[5]

A recent article in the *Lancet* provides a vivid illustration of the complexity to which Dr. Garland alludes.[12] The opening lines of the article are designed to capture our attention: "There are no safe drugs. Adverse reactions are always a potential hazard and the problem is magnified when additional drugs are used." The title of the article suggests the nature of the author's concern and a modest aid for the harried physician: "The Drug Disc: Warning System for Drug Interactions." "Today," they argue, "so many drugs are available for general use that it is becoming increasingly difficult for the practicing physician to sustain such a mass of detailed information. The drug disc (which is a system for anticipating dangerous combinations as well as decreased or increased effects in particular combinations) attempts to overcome this problem by a simple and portable system, thereby avoiding many of the hazards implicit in the use of drug combinations."[12] I am not competent to evaluate the usefulness of the drug disc described; I mention it only as an illustration of a problem.

My brief practical education in clinical pharmacology has impressed me with the continuing risk and uncertainty of drug prescription and, given the current state of knowledge, the high probability of an essential, presumably necessary, pragmatism which is nonetheless risky for the patient. Pharmacological management of the elderly patient is an especially important aspect of this general problem.

When the problems of drugs for the elderly have been discussed during the past decade, economic issues have been featured more frequently than therapeutic issues. Not long ago the high cost of drugs was stressed, but this concern has been dissipated somewhat by the higher cost of every other aspect of health care. More recently, the Senate Special Committee on Aging has probed suspect arrangements between nursing homes and pharmacists and hinted darkly that if the drug schedules appearing on the books of some nursing homes are accurate, the residents of those nursing homes are probably overmedicated.[11]

The concerns are real but they mask a more basic problem: The case of drugs in the therapeutic management of elderly patients is uninformed by definitive information. It is my impression that the pharmacological management of the elderly patient is among the least understood aspects of clinical pharmacology and that little is currently being done to correct this deficiency.

This impression is admittedly that of a layman in pharmacology. But let me comment on how this impression emerged. First, I have yet to meet a medical clinician who expressed confidence in his knowledge of the use of drugs in the management of his elderly patients or who believed that the elderly patient presented no special problems.

Second, I have encountered time and again the belief among clinicians that, given the high frequency of multiple-drug administration to elderly patients, the incidence of "problems of medical progress" is high. I cannot cite the evidence that this is so, but then, I am not aware that the issue has ever been studied carefully.

Third, in preparation of this article, I scanned a number of well-known sources of information about pharmacology for medical clinicians. Consider, for example, Walter Modell's *Drugs of Choice*. In all editions through the current one (1972-1973), the only chapter that considers age is devoted to children, and the index makes no reference at all to "age" or "aging."[7] Out of curiosity, I wrote Dr. Modell expressing surprise at the omission of a chapter on problems of drugs for and drug management of the elderly patient. In reply, Dr. Modell wrote:

> The question has not escaped me but the solution has. I have been considering it for some time and what has stopped me is that I find so little hard information on the subject, so little that is not merely obvious generalization. Nevertheless, we will have a chapter

on it in the next edition, but one. In preparing for this we are dropping the chapter on the choice of drugs for children in the 1974-75 edition. The next edition will have a single chapter relating drug choice to all age groups. If you have any suggestions, I would be glad to have them.[8]

Dr. Modell's last sentence poses a challenge and an opportunity. What do we know about drugs and the elderly? What ought we to know?

I hope that this volume will be a modest and useful beginning in answering these important questions.

* * *

There is a happy postscript to be added to the hopeful conclusion of my 1974 statement. Subsequent editions of Modell's *Drugs of Choice* have included a chapter on drug use with specific reference to late life.

In balance, it should be clear that I am not disinterested in substance abuse *by* older people. I am simply more disturbed about substance abuse in which older people are the unwitting victims. We ought to reduce such abuse. We can. We must.

REFERENCES

1. Eimerl, T. S.: The pattern of prescribing. *College Gen Practitioners J*, 5:468-479, 1962.
2. Eisdorfer, C. and Fann, W. E. (Eds.): *Psychopharmacology and Aging*. New York, Plenum Pr, 1973.
3. Fann, W. E. and Maddox, G. L. (Eds.): *Drug Issues in Geropsychiatry*. Baltimore, Williams & Wilkins, 1974.
4. Goodman, L.: The problem of drug efficacy: An exercise in dissection. In Talalay, P. (Ed.): *Drugs in Our Society*. Baltimore, Johns Hopkins, 1964.
5. Garland, J.: Dissemination of information on drugs to the physician. In Talalay, P. (Ed.): *Drugs in Our Society*. Baltimore, Johns Hopkins, 1964.
6. Lennard, H. L., Epstein, L., and Rosenthal, M.: The methadone illusion. *Science*, 176:881-884, 1972.
7. Modell, W.: *Drugs of Choice* (consecutive editions). St. Louis, Mosby, 1958-1972.
8. Modell, W.: Drugs and the older patient. Personal communication with the author, 1973.

9. Rensberger, B.: Thousands a year killed by faulty prescriptions. *New York Times, 125*: (Jan. 28, 1976), pp. 1, 17.
10. U.S. Department of Health, Education and Welfare: *Medical Malpractice: Report of the Secretary's Commission on Medical Malpractice.* Washington, D.C., U.S. Govt Print Office, 1973.
11. U.S. Senate Special Committee on Aging: *Drugs in Nursing Homes: Misuse, High Costs and Kickbacks.* Washington, D.C., U.S. Govt Print Office, Jan., 1975.
12. Whiting, B., Goldberg, A., and Waldie, P.: The drug disc: Warning system for drug interactions. *Lancet, 1*:1037-1038, 12 May, 1973.

Chapter 2

DRUGS AND THE ELDERLY*

FRANK J. WHITTINGTON, PH.D.
DAVID M. PETERSEN, PH.D.

THE ABUSE AND MISUSE of drugs is a social phenomenon which has, in this century, grown into one of the most common and troublesome problems in American society. Although drug abuse is found at all age-levels, the elderly drug user has rarely been studied. References to drug abuse problems among older persons are abundant, particularly in the geriatric and pharmacological literature, but there appears to be little systematic research on the use or misuse of drugs (other than alcohol) among this group. What little there is has been completed very recently.[3, 8, 9, 18, 23]

It is not surprising that little research has been done on older drug abusers and addicts, as adolescents and young adults have greatly increased their drug use since World War II. Another reason that drug use among the elderly has commanded so little attention is that drug researchers and clinicians have long believed that the drug abuser either dies an early death or "matures out" of his addiction in his later years.[28] One final possibility has to do with the generally devalued social status occupied by the elderly in this society. Aside from the covert nature of many geriatric drug problems, there has been a much greater tendency on the part of researchers and clinicians to overlook and discount the importance of drug misuse among the elderly.

In this chapter, relevant literature and available research

---

* Revised version of "Drug Use Among the Elderly: A Review," *Journal of Psychedelic Drugs*, 9:(January/March, 1977), 25-37. Reprinted by permission of STASH Press, 118 S. Bedford St., Madison, Wisconsin 53703.

evidence on drug use and misuse among the elderly is reviewed and summarized. Gaps in this literature and research and suggestions of specific research problems that need to be addressed are identified. The reader is alerted to the fact that the literature under review reflects a methodological problem which has long plagued drug researchers; namely, that no standard definition of drug use or misuse exists. This is hardly surprising, however, since these materials have been written by persons from such diverse disciplinary orientations as medicine, psychiatry, pharmacology, psychology, sociology, and social work. It must be noted, then, that direct comparison between the findings of these various studies is often impossible, but the relevant aspects of each report are synopsized in Table 2-I to facilitate such scrutiny.

USE OF LEGAL DRUGS

The literature on drug use and misuse is conventionally divided into two broad categories: that dealing with legal drugs and that concerned with illegal drugs. Consequently, patterns of both the use and misuse of legal drugs are discussed first and then the abuse of illegal drugs.

Contrary to the age-pattern of alcohol use, older people use far more drugs per capita than do younger people. Although the elderly constitute only 10 percent of the population, the Task Force on Prescription Drugs in their publication *The Drug Users*[25] reports that they received roughly one fourth of all prescriptions written in 1967, and it is probably safe to assume that their share of the over-the-counter drug market was at least as large. The Task Force also noted that the average person over age sixty-five acquired about three times as many prescribed drugs and spent about three times as much for their drugs as those under the age of sixty-five.

The conditions for which drugs were most commonly prescribed for the elderly in 1966 were, in order of frequency, the following: heart disease, hypertension, arthritis and rheumatism, and mental and nervous conditions. Of all drugs prescribed for elderly persons, the four therapeutic categories most frequently prescribed were as follows: cardiovascular medicines (22%),

TABLE 2-I
STUDIES OF DRUG USE AMONG THE ELDERLY

Study	Type of Substance	Sample	Site of Data Collection	Findings
Ball and Chambers (1970)	Opiates	2,932 addict patients	U.S. Public Health Service Hospitals, Lexington, KY and Fort Worth, TX	10 percent of all admissions during 1963 were persons aged 50 and over
Ball and Lau (1966)	Opiates	137 Chinese male addict patients	U.S. Public Health Service Hospital, Lexington, KY	Almost 90 percent (88.4%) were over 40 years of age and most were long-term addicts
Barton and Hurst (1966)	Tranquilizers	53 geriatric patients	Psychiatric hospital	The majority of elderly demented patients receiving tranquilizers showed no significant deterioration when medication removed (average age = 76)
Capel and Stewart (1971) and Capel et al. (1972)	Opiates	38 addicts	New Orleans, LA	In addition to those older addicts enrolled in the New Orleans methadone maintenance program, 38 addicts were identified in the community who were not in any treatment program
Chambers (1971)	Seventeen categories of psychoactive drugs	7,500 persons	Seventeen regions of New York State	The oldest age-group (50 and over) was found to have the largest percentage of regular users of barbiturates, nonbarbiturate sedative-hypnotics, minor and major tranquilizers
Kastenbaum et al. (1964)	Thioridazine (tranquilizer) and dextroamphetamine (stimulant)	27 geriatric patients	Geriatric hospital in Framingham, MA	No systematic evidence was found for improvement in cognitive functioning due to the administration of either drug
Learoyd (1972)	Psychotropic drugs	236 patients	North Ryde Psychiatric Centre, New South Wales, Australia	16 percent of all admissions presented disorders directly attributable to the ill effects of psychoactive drugs

TABLE 2-I (Continued)

Study	Type of Substance	Sample	Site of Data Collection	Findings
Milliren (1977)	Tranquilizers	131 geriatric patients	Long-term care facility for the elderly	Females are more likely than males to receive tranquilizers; among males, low mental status and judged unfriendliness to the staff led to the administration of tranquilizers
O'Donnell (1969)	Opiates	266 former addict patients	U.S. Public Health Service Hospital, Lexington, KY	Follow-up study revealed that only 21 addicts remained addicted to narcotics
Pascarelli (1972) and Pascarelli and Fischer (1974)	Methadone	320 methadone patients	Roosevelt Hospital, Methadone Maintenance Program, New York City	2 percent of all patients were found to be over 60
Pescor (1942)	Opiates	47 addict physicians	U.S. Public Health Service Hospital, Fort Worth, TX	The typical addict physician was 52, married, living in a small town, engaged in general practice, and addicted to morphine
Petersen and Thomas (1975)	Ten categories of legal and illegal drugs	60 emergency room patients	Jackson Memorial Hospital, Miami, FL	Older patients (50 and over) treated for acute drug reactions constituted 5.4 percent of all admissions
Winick (1961)	Opiates	98 addict physicians	Six northeastern states	These addicts ranged in age between 28 and 78 with a mean age of 44; most were married, general practitioners, living in large cities, using meperidine instead of morphine
Winick (1962)	Opiates	7,234 addicts	Federal Bureau of Narcotics "Active Addict" list	Many addicts originally reported in 1955 had disappeared from the files by 1960; that most were between the ages of 35-45 led to the suggestion of a "burn-out" hypothesis

tranquilizers (10%), diuretics (9%), and sedative-hypnotics (9%). Although mental and nervous conditions account for less than 7 percent of all prescriptions written, four psychotropic substances, chlordiazepoxide (Librium®), glutethimide (Doriden®), phenobarbital (Luminal®), and diazepam (Valium®), are among the ten most prescribed drugs for persons sixty-five and over.[25]

Although no data comparable to that found in the national survey of drinking practices[7] exists for drug use, one statewide survey has been completed. Although the Chambers[10] survey was designed to assess only drug use and did not specifically address drug misuse or abuse, by definition in contemporary American society, reported use of illegal substances, e.g. heroin or cocaine, constitutes abuse. The Chambers survey assessed incidence, prevalence, and extent of use of seventeen categories of psychoactive drugs and found several relationships between age and regular use of such drugs. The oldest age-group (fifty years and over) was found to have the largest percentage of regular users of barbiturate sedative-hypnotics (Luminal or Seconal®), 58 percent; nonbarbiturate sedative-hypnotics (Doriden or Placidyl®), 58 percent; minor tranquilizers (Valium or Librium), 42 percent; and major tranquilizers (Thorazine® or Mellaril®), 48 percent. A bimodal age-relationship was discovered for two other drug categories; regular users of amphetamines (Dexedrine® or Benzedrine®) as well as noncontrolled narcotics and prescription non-narcotic analgesics (Talwin® or Darvon®) were concentrated about equally in the eighteen to twenty-four and over-fifty age-groups. As might be expected, however, the regular use of marijuana, LSD, other psychotogens (mescaline or psilocybin), methedrine, heroin, and cocaine is strongly associated with younger age-groups with almost no usage in the over-fifty age-group. Finally, there appeared to be no relationship between age and regular use of antidepressants (Elavil® or Tofranil®), diet pills (Dexamyl® or Preludin®), or controlled opium derivatives other than heroin (morphine or codeine), with such use being about evenly distributed among the age-groups.

MISUSE OF LEGAL DRUGS

Since the elderly evidence substantially higher rates of drug consumption than others in society and are therefore more at risk, it seems quite likely that they should also have higher rates of misuse or abuse. Unfortunately, there is very little official data to support this assumption. Nationwide data reported to the United States Department of Justice through the Drug Abuse Warning Network (DAWN) program from such medical sources as hospitals and emergency rooms indicate that in the first half of 1973, people over fifty were involved in 6 percent of the reported total drug incidents with barbiturate sedatives, tranquilizers, and alcohol-other drug interactions.[14]

These data are consistent with a study by Petersen and Thomas,[23] who found that older patients (fifty years and over) treated in a hospital emergency room for acute drug reactions (overdoses) constituted only 5 percent of the total sample of overdose patients seen at that hospital. Thus, older people are somewhat underrepresented among drug users who seek emergency medical care for their drug-induced reactions. Petersen and Thomas note, however, that many drug reactions are probably never presented in a clinical setting and are probably being managed elsewhere in other ways. Thus, the real dimensions of this phenomenon can still only be estimated.

There is, however, a definite relationship between the use and misuse of specific drugs resulting in an acute drug reaction. Although more than 20 percent of the younger patients in the Petersen and Thomas study who experienced an acute drug reaction had misused an illicit substance, *none* of the older patients had done so; all admissions of those over age fifty resulted from an acute reaction to a legally available drug. Over 80 percent of all acute drug reactions involved the misuse of a psychotropic (either a sedative or a tranquilizer), primarily Valium, Tuinal®, and Luminal, and an additional 10 percent resulted from the misuse of the non-narcotic analgesic Darvon. Thus, although available evidence suggests that, compared to younger persons, the older drug abuser is underrepresented among those who come to public attention, their drug misuse does seem to result from those drugs most often prescribed for them.

There is some evidence that nursing homes and other geriatric facilities may contribute directly to the misuse of drugs by the elderly. In many instances, these institutions elicit and often continue indefinitely a physician's prescription for control drugs that may have no therapeutic function other than to aid in the management of difficult patients.[17, 18, 26] Barton and Hurst,[3] for example, studied the effects of chlorpromazine (Thorazine), a major tranquilizer, on a group of institutionalized elderly women and found that the drug gave little if any symptomatic relief. They concluded that some 80 percent of aged mental patients are receiving tranquilizers unnecessarily. Although these findings are not undisputed,[11] Kastenbaum, Slater, and Aisenberg[15] found no systematic evidence for improvement of cognitive functioning among a sample of hospitalized geriatric patients due to the administration of either a tranquilizer (Mellaril) or a stimulant (Dexedrine).

Concerning the misuse of drugs among the elderly, there is a series of problems that can be directly tied to the effects of the aging process itself. Although, as with the young drug abuser, many problems are the result of excessive self-medication or other inappropriate use, a considerable amount of attention has recently been directed to the effect of the aging process on pharmacological efficacy and safety. Specifically, interest has centered on drug interactions, side effects, and long-term drug management for the elderly.[12, 13, 16] For example, in elderly patients with multiple chronic conditions for which different drugs are being ingested concurrently, drug interactions are extremely likely occurrences. As Learoyd[17] points out, older patients metabolize drugs more slowly than younger persons, and when two are taken simultaneously, each can have a potentiating effect on the other, thus heightening the risk of drug intoxification. Moreover, many drugs produce side effects—physical, emotional, or both—which must be anticipated, and for many reasons, such side effects are more common and often more severe in elderly patients.[16] Thus, health care professionals concerned with problems of the aged have become increasingly aware that the elderly may experience drug-related problems not attributable to misuse on their part.

ABUSE OF NARCOTIC DRUGS

Although a wide variety of drugs are classified as illegal, the paucity of data regarding use of these substances necessitates limiting discussion in this section to opiate abuse. It is well known that the most visible opiate addicts in the United States are young adults. Incidence data for all patients admitted to the United States Public Health Service Hospital in Lexington, Kentucky, in 1963, for example, revealed that 80 percent of the admissions for that year were under forty years of age, while only slightly more than 10 percent were persons fifty years and over. Those over sixty years comprised less than 4 percent of those admitted during that year.[1] The question of why relatively few known addicts are older than forty has interested a number of investigators.

Winick,[28] analyzing the Active Addict list of the Federal Bureau of Narcotics, noticed that many addicts disappeared from the files between the ages of thirty-five and forty-five. This observation led him to hypothesize a *maturing-out process* resulting in a cessation of addiction due either to the addict's chronological age or to the length of time he has been addicted. Winick believes that most addicts are hooked during their late teens or early twenties when their emotional problems with sexuality, aggressiveness, and occupational choice are most severe. Some of these addicts, he suggests, may reach a point of *emotional homeostasis* during their thirties when life stress may be reduced enough so they can deal with their problems without relying on drugs. Others simply "burn out" of their addiction, i.e. they die or become too debilitated to supply their habits.

There is evidence, however, that the maturing-out hypothesis may not be valid, at least for many addicts. O'Donnell's[19] follow-up study of 266 former patients of the Lexington Hospital demonstrates the weaknesses inherent in the use of the Bureau of Narcotics' master file of drug addicts to do this sort of research. Of these former patients, 144 had died, and only 21 were found to be still addicted to narcotics. The remainder were either addicted to other drugs, institutionalized, or abstinent. However, of the 21 addicts, only *one* was found to have ever been on the Bureau's list of active addicts; all of the others either were unknown to the Bureau, were classified as "medical" addicts, or had been suspected of being addicts but, due to lack of evidence, were never formally listed. This finding does not in itself disprove Winick's maturing-out thesis, but there is mounting evidence that a substantial number of older addicts do exist, whether they come to official attention or not.

At least two special addict groups have been identified which tend to be older than the overall addict population. The first is composed of Chinese-American opium addicts, most of whom became addicted early in this century after immigrating to this country from China. The Ball and Lau[2] study of a group of Chinese addicts released from the federal addiction treatment center in Lexington between 1957 and 1962 revealed that 88.4 percent were over forty years of age and that most were long-term addicts, having begun using narcotics before age thirty. This addict cohort is quickly disappearing, however, and very few new addicts are appearing among the second and third generations of Chinese-Americans. It is assumed that the native-born Chinese were acculturated and failed to continue the opium tradition. Yet, because of this link between drug use and ethnic subculture, in addition to their advanced age, this addict group is of particular interest.

Another addict group much older than average is that of physician narcotic addicts. With an estimated addiction rate (1%) thirty times that of the general population, physicians present a much different pattern of drug abuse than the usual addict. An early study by Pescor[22] found them to be typically older (average age fifty-two), married, small-town, general practitioners who began using morphine about age thirty-nine to relieve pain. Twenty years later, Winick[27] studied a slightly younger group of addict physicians who ranged between twenty-eight and seventy-eight years old, with a mean age of forty-four. Again, most were married general practitioners, but this sample lived mainly in large cities, and almost all (80%) used meperidine (Demerol®) instead of morphine. More important, however, was the finding that, with respect to their reasons for becoming addicted, these physicians were much more similar to other addicts than those described by Pescor. According to Winick,[27] "These physicians appear to have been addiction-prone through some combination of role strain, passivity, omnipotence, and effects of the drug." Thus, personality and reality factors were more salient than a medically related influence such as pain.

Two more recent studies give further indication that older

addicts do exist, even if hidden from official eyes. In an investigation of narcotic addicts in New Orleans, Capel and Stewart[9] and Capel et al.[8] discovered a substantial number of addicts between the ages of forty-five and seventy-five. In addition to identifying approximately sixty addicts over forty-five years of age involved in a methadone maintenance program (about 5% of the total), these researchers were also able to find thirty-eight addicts in the community not in any treatment program. Contrary to the burn-out or mature-out hypotheses, these older addicts had not ceased using opiates but had succeeded in camouflaging their habits through a variety of adaptive techniques, thus avoiding official scrutiny and harassment. By relying primarily on the neighborhood pusher, by switching from a more scarce, less dependable drug, such as heroin, to a cheaper, more easily obtainable drug, such as Dilaudid®, by adjusting to a decreased daily intake or to a barbiturate or alcohol substitute on occasion, these older, streetwise addicts were managing their habits more or less unnoticed by authorities and certainly without benefit of treatment.

Pascarelli's[20] observation of the older patients in a methadone maintenance program at Roosevelt Hospital in New York City appears to bear out Capel's findings. Although addicts over sixty presently constitute only about 0.5 percent of the 34,000 methadone patients in New York City, they accounted for over 2 percent of the addicts in the Roosevelt program. Pascarelli argues that this figure is probably a serious underestimate of the size of the older addict population. He depicts the older addict as one who presents a low profile in the community by using the same adaptive techniques described above. In addition, elderly users are the least satisfied with methadone treatment and, once in the program, are the least likely to request detoxification. This dissatisfaction, coupled with an ability to manage the habit relatively well in the community, probably steers many older addicts away from treatment. Yet, judging by the number of middle-aged addicts now in treatment, Pascarelli and Fischer[21] expect the older addict group to increase markedly over the next two decades. They base their prediction on the fact that 34 percent of their treatment population is already over forty and, as they age, will cause both absolute and relative growth of the older addict group. This percentage is, however, somewhat higher than the 20 percent in 1963 reported for the Lexington population[1] and more than double the Capel and Stewart[9] estimate that one-eighth of the New Orleans addict population was over forty. These discrepancies are difficult to explain with certainty because they may reflect age differences in help-seeking behavior, in treatment modality sought, and/or in geographic location. Yet, even on the assumption of a relatively low addict population over forty, Capel and Stewart[9] estimate that ". . . by 1980 New Orleans can anticipate that its citizens over 65 will include some 150 additional mainline narcotic addicts . . . each year."

DISCUSSION

With the preponderant involvement of youth in drug use and misuse in the United States, it is not surprising that the majority of the writing and research in this area has dealt with younger people. Literature indicating that drug misuse among the elderly is a growing problem is of recent date but has been appearing with increasing regularity.[4, 6, 14, 24, 29] In our review of the literature it was found that a wide variety of issues have been addressed by the authors, including the reasons for drug abuse in the aging, factors that exacerbate elderly drug misuse, and suggestions for action. Despite a rather substantial and still-growing literature, our review found very little empirical basis for the discussion of these topics. Although a number of drug-related issues have been raised regarding drug use among the elderly, other than in geriatric pharmacology, very little basic or applied research has been conducted in this area. In our opinion, this lack of research data represents a fundamental problem for health care professionals, social gerontologists, and others concerned with misuse of drugs by older persons.

Available data certainly suggest that the elderly are the largest consumers of certain drugs and, moreover, are at high risk as to the potential misuse of these substances. Yet, basic data on the real extent of use and misuse of psychoactive drugs by older people are lacking. Although some comparative data relevant to these issues are available from larger investigations, no single study as yet has focused on the incidence and prevalence of drug use and misuse among older persons. In addition, the underlying causes of drug abuse and dependency among older persons is an area that has not yet been researched. Lacking are such basic data as the demographic and social correlates (sex, race, education, social position), the behavioral correlates (type and context of and reasons for use), and the personal correlates (health and personality characteristics of users, attitudes toward drug use, effects of use) of drug use and misuse among the elderly. For example, it is often assumed, but not yet demonstrated, that older women are the primary misusers of psychoactive drugs, that older drug misusers are likely to be in poor physical and mental condition, and that misuse generally comes to the attention of health authorities. It is even suggested that older and younger persons may sometimes misuse drugs for similar reasons, including the lack of meaningful work opportunities or leisure time pursuits, boredom, and loneliness. Yet, the fact is that there are no data to support any of these assertions.

Existing data suggest that the various facilities of the health care system (hospitals, geriatric institutions, mental health clinics, and so on) are not receiving many elderly persons for substance abuse problems. Are there significant numbers of elderly drug abusers hidden in the community, as some suggest? If so, why do they not come to the attention of the existing health care facilities? Is it because they are generally reluctant to seek help, or are they able to manage their problems in the community without professional help?

Little is known concerning the responses of elderly patients to treatment for drug-related problems. Research would suggest that those over forty tend to respond more favorably than younger persons to treatment intervention for alcohol problems.[5] Moreover, although the early results with alcohol are promising, there is little information regarding the effective use of psychoactive drugs in the management and treatment of elderly patients, and there is even some data indicating that many drugs are ineffectively and unnecessarily administered.

Finally, elderly drug abusers deserve more research attention, both to increase basic knowledge about them and to assist in providing them with meaningful programs of treatment and social rehabilitation.

REFERENCES

1. Ball, J. C. and Chambers, C. D.: *The Epidemiology of Opiate Addiction in the United States.* Springfield, Thomas, 1970.
2. Ball, J. C. and Lau, M. P.: The Chinese narcotic addict in the United States. *Soc Forces,* 45:68-72, 1966.
3. Barton, R. and Hurst, L.: Unnecessary use of tranquilizers in elderly patients. *Br J Psychiatry,* 112:989-990, 1966.
4. Basen, M. M.: The elderly and drugs—Problem overview and program strategy. *Public Health Rep,* 92:43-48, 1977.
5. Bateman, N. I. and Petersen, D. M.: Factors related to outcome of treatment for hospitalized white male and female alcoholics. *J Drug Issues,* 2:66-74, 1972.
6. Bourne, P. G.: Drug abuse in the aging. *Perspect Aging,* 2:18-20, 1973.
7. Cahalan, D., Cisin, I. H., and Crossley, H. M.: *American Drinking Practices.* New Brunswick, New Jersey, Rutgers U Pr, 1969.
8. Capel, W. C., Goldsmith, B. M., Waddell, K. J., and Stewart, G. T.: The aging narcotic addict: An increasing problem for the next decades. *J Gerontol,* 27:102-106, 1972.
9. Capel, W. C. and Stewart, G. T.: The management of drug abuse in aging populations: New Orleans findings. *J Drug Issues,* 1:114-121, 1971.
10. Chambers, C. D.: *An Assessment of Drug Use in the General Population.* New York, New York State Narcotic Addiction Control Commission, 1971.
11. Daniel, R.: Psychiatric drug use and abuse in the aged. *Geriatrics,* 25:144-158, 1970.
12. Davis, R. H. and Smith, W. K. (Eds.): *Drugs and the Elderly.* Los Angeles, Ethel Percy Andrus Gerontology Center, U of S Cal, 1973.
13. Fann, W. E. and Maddox, G. L. (Eds.): *Drug Issues in Geropsychiatry.* Baltimore, Williams & Wilkins, 1974.
14. Heller, F. J. and Wynne, R.: Drug misuse by the elderly: Indications and treatment suggestions. In Senay, E., Shorty, V., and Alksne, H. (Eds.): *Developments in the Field of Drug Abuse.* Cambridge, Massachusetts, Schenkman, 1975.
15. Kastenbaum, R., Slater, P. E., and Aisenberg, R.: Toward a conceptual model of geriatric psychopharmacology: An experiment with thioridazine and dextro-amphetamine. *Gerontologist,* 4:68-71, 1964.
16. Lamy, P. P. and Kitler, M. E.: Drugs and the geriatric patient. *J Am Geriatr Soc,* 19:23-33, 1971.
17. Learoyd, B. M.: Psychotropic drugs and the elderly patient. *Med J Aust,* 1:1131-1133, 1972.
18. Milliren, J. W.: Some contingencies affecting the utilization of tranquilizers in long-term care of the elderly. *J Health Soc Behav,* 18:206-211, 1977.

19. O'Donnell, J. A.: *Narcotic Addicts in Kentucky.* Washington, D.C., Public Health Service Publ. No. 1881, U.S. Govt Print Office, 1969.
20. Pascarelli, E.: Alcoholism and drug addiction in the elderly. *Geriatr Focus, 11*:1, 4-5, 1972.
21. Pascarelli, E. F. and Fischer, W.: Drug dependence in the elderly. *Int J Aging Human Dev, 5*:347-356, 1974.
22. Pescor, M. J.: Physician drug addicts. *Dis Nerv Syst, 3*:173-174, 1942.
23. Petersen, D. M. and Thomas, C. W.: Acute drug reactions among the elderly. *J Gerontol, 30*:552-556, 1975.
24. Schuckit, M. A.: Geriatric alcoholism and drug abuse. *Gerontologist, 17*:168-174, 1977.
25. Task Force on Prescription Drugs: *The Drug Users.* Washington, D.C., U.S. Govt Print Office, 1968.
26. Townsend, C.: *Old Age: The Last Segregation.* New York, Grossman, 1971.
27. Winick, C.: Physician narcotic addicts. *Soc Prob, 9*:174-186, 1961.
28. ———: Maturing out of addiction. *Bull Narc, 14*:1-7, 1962.
29. Wynne, R. D. and Heller, F.: Drug overuse among the elderly: A growing problem. *Perspect Aging, 2*:15-18, 1973.

Chapter 3

ALCOHOL AND THE ELDERLY

SHELDON ZIMBERG, M.D.

IT HAS BEEN commonly accepted that alcohol abuse is not a significant problem among the elderly. Considerable evidence has accumulated in recent years, however, which suggests that the old as well as the young use and misuse alcohol in significant numbers. The purpose of this chapter is to review the available data regarding this drug problem among the elderly (*see* Table 3-I for a synopsis of the empirical studies).

EPIDEMIOLOGY OF ALCOHOL USE

Cahalan, Cisin, and Crossley[4] in their national survey of drinking behavior and attitudes found that heavy drinking declines substantially in both sexes after age forty-nine and observed an even greater drop in men after age sixty-four. Studies of psychiatric hospital admissions and outpatient clinic admissions suggest the age incidence of alcoholism peaks between the ages of thirty-five and fifty and experiences a decline in incidence with increasing age above fifty.[12, 15, 16]

There seems to be a substantial amount of attrition in the natural course of alcoholism. Alcoholism tends to shorten the life span of individuals and results in higher death rates for cardiovascular disorders, pneumonia, cirrhosis of the liver, accidents, and suicide.[18, 20] Cahalan and his associates[4] noted significantly more individuals had had a drinking problem in the past than did during the three-year period they studied, which suggests the possibility of a significant rate of spontaneous remission of alcoholism. Drew[8] presented data which also suggested that, rather than a tendency for alcoholics to die at an earlier age and regardless of the effects of treatment, alcoholism is a self-limiting disease and remits spontaneously with advancing age. Therefore, a considerable body of evidence exists that supports the commonly held belief that alcohol abuse is not a significant problem among the elderly. However, other evidence indicates that alcohol abuse is in fact a serious problem among elderly people but one that may well be underdiagnosed and underreported.

In a household-alcoholism prevalence survey using probability sampling techniques conducted in the Washington Heights area of Manhattan,[1] it was noted that the peak prevalence of alcoholism occurred in the forty-five-to-fifty-four-year age-group at 23 per 1,000 population aged twenty years and over. Although prevalence decreased to 17 per 1,000 for the age-group fifty-five to sixty-five years, there was a second peak prevalence of 22 per 1,000 at the sixty-five-to-seventy-four-year age-group and then a drop to 12 per 1,000 for the seventy-five-and-over age-group.

A probability sample of members of the United Automobile Workers Union twenty-one years of age and over was conducted in the Baltimore metropolitan area during 1973.[22] This study found that among men aged sixty and over, 65 percent of the drinkers in the sample were heavy drinkers, and 10 percent were heavy-escape drinkers. The heavy-escape drinkers were considered alcoholics in this study. Among the women drinkers aged sixty and over, 40 percent were heavy drinkers, and 20 percent were heavy-escape drinkers. These older women had the highest alcoholism rate of any age-group studied, either women or men.

In addition to the prevalence studies, there is other evidence that alcoholism is a significant geriatric problem. In a study of 534 patients over age sixty admitted to a psychiatric observation ward in San Francisco General Hospital, Simon, Epstein, and Reynolds[23] found that 28 percent had a "serious drinking problem." Of these, 5 percent were heavy drinkers, but their drinking had not played an important role in their hospitalization. The other 23 percent were classified as alcoholics whose alcoholism caused or was implicated in their hospitalization. Also in San Francisco, Epstein, Mills, and Simon[10] found that, of 722 individuals aged sixty and over arrested for minor crimes by the

TABLE 3-I
STUDIES OF ALCOHOL USE AMONG THE ELDERLY

Study	Type of Substance	Sample	Site of Data Collection	Findings
Bailey et al. (1965)	Alcohol	3,959 dwelling units	Washington Heights Health District, New York City	A second peak rate for alcoholism was found for those persons aged 65-74
Becker and Cesar (1973)	Beer	32 geriatric patients	Hospital psychiatric ward, Norristown State Hospital, Norristown, PA	Elderly psychiatric patients (average age = 69) given beer showed greater social interaction than those patients who did not receive this beverage, while ward behavior of neither patient group was improved
Cahalan et al. (1969)	Alcohol	2,746 persons	Households throughout the United States	The percentage of abstainers from alcohol use was highest among those persons over 60
Chien et al. (1973)	Alcohol, doxepin (an antidepressant) and other psychotropic medications	64 nursing home patients	Two nursing homes located in Boston, MA	Alcohol was associated with significant improvement in all experimental groups regardless of the setting in which it was administered and no group showed improvement while under drug therapy
Epstein et al. (1970)	Alcohol	722 elderly offenders	San Francisco, CA	Over 80 percent of all arrests of persons aged 60 and over were for drunkenness
Gorwitz et al. (1970)	Alcohol	6,432 alcoholic patients	Mental health facilities throughout the state of Maryland	Age incidence of alcoholism was found to peak between the ages 35-50
Locke et al. (1960)	Alcohol	1,778 alcoholic patients	Ohio State mental hospitals	Age incidence of alcoholism was found to peak between the ages of 35-50
Malzberg (1947)	Alcohol	675 alcoholic patients	New York State mental hospitals	Age incidence of alcoholism was found to peak between the ages of 35-50

TABLE 3-I (Continued)

Study	Type of Substance	Sample	Site of Data Collection	Findings
McCusker et al. (1971)	Alcohol	118 patients	Harlem Hospital, New York City	63 percent of the males and 35 percent of the females in the 50-69 age group were alcoholics
Schuckit and Miller (1975)	Alcohol	113 male alcoholic patients	Medical wards at La Jolla Veterans Administration Hospital	Among admissions 65 years and over, 18 percent were classified as alcoholic
Siassi et al. (1973)	Alcohol	937 persons	United Automobile Workers Union, Baltimore, MD	Among men age 60 and over, 65 percent of the drinkers were classified as heavy drinkers, and 10 percent as heavy-escape drinkers or alcoholics
Simon et al. (1968)	Alcohol	534 hospital patients	San Francisco General Hospital, San Francisco, CA	28 percent of these patients 60 and older had a serious drinking problem at the time of their admission
Zimberg (1969)	Alcohol	35 geriatric patients	Geriatric Psychiatry Outpatient Program, Harlem Community, New York City	Of all patients seen in the first year of operation of this program, 12 percent were noted to have an alcoholism problem
Zimberg (1971)	Alcohol	24 medical patients	Private dwellings in Harlem Community, New York City	13 percent of the patients in a home care program were diagnosed as having an alcoholism problem
Zimberg (1974)	Alcohol	1,636 medical patients	Mental Health Center, Suburban Rockland County, NY	Of all patient admissions during the first six months of 1972, 87 (5.3%) were 65 years of age and over; 17 percent of these patients had an alcohol abuse problem upon admission

San Francisco Police, 82.3 percent were charged with drunkenness—a much higher proportion than that in any other age-group. Therefore, at least in San Francisco, many elderly people are admitted to psychiatric hospitals for alcoholism, and many others are arrested by the police for public intoxication.

A prevalence study of patients newly admitted to the medical wards of Harlem Hospital Center in New York City was conducted by McCusker, Cherubin, and Zimberg.[17] This study found that 63 percent of the men and 35 percent of the women in the fifty-to-sixty-nine-year-old age-group were alcoholics. In the age-group seventy and over, five of the nine male patients were alcoholic, but none of the women. Schuckit and Miller[21] conducted a survey of admissions of patients sixty-five years of age and over to the acute medical wards of a California Veterans Administration Hospital and found that 18 percent of the patients were alcoholic. Thus, elderly alcoholics come to the attention of inpatient medical services as well as psychiatric programs.

An alcoholism problem was noted by Zimberg in his work with the elderly in the Harlem community in a geriatric psychiatry outpatient program.[25] In this program, 12 percent of the patients seen in the first year of operation were noted to have an alcoholism problem. As consultant to a medical home care program in Harlem,[26] Zimberg observed that 13 percent of the patients he visited had an alcoholism problem.

The problem of alcoholism among the elderly is not a problem confined to urban areas. At a federally funded community mental health center in suburban Rockland County, New York, there were, during the first six months of 1972, 1,636 patients admitted, 87 of whom (5.3%) were sixty-five years of age and over. It was noted that 17 percent of these patients had an alcohol abuse problem upon admission.[27]

Carruth and his associates[5] interviewed staff members of health, social service, and criminal justice agencies in three communities, representing urban, rural, and an urban-rural population mix, regarding the extent of problem drinking among their elderly clients. They found that 95 percent of these respondents had seen an older problem drinker as a client in the last year. They also noted that the alcoholism information and referral services that they surveyed reported that 30 percent of all calls came from persons over the age of fifty-five.

Although the true prevalence of alcoholism among the elderly has not been documented and there are serious disagreements about the significance of this problem, several factors in relation to alcohol consumption and the aging process should be considered. The work of deLint[7] and discussion of his work by Faris[11] suggests that the frequency distribution of alcohol consumption in a population can be determined and that it occurs in a log normal curve distribution. That is, the more alcohol that is consumed per capita, the more alcoholics there will be in a population, and, conversely, the less alcohol consumed per capita, the fewer alcoholics there will be. Current consumption rates in the United States are rising rapidly and, therefore, if deLint is correct, we can expect more alcoholism.

The fact that people are living longer and the fact that services for the elderly are greatly lacking contribute to increasing psychological, social, and physical problems the elderly are facing. Such problems with a rising per capita consumption of alcohol may lead to an increase in alcohol abuse problems in the elderly. In any case, this issue is an important one and should have further study in regard to attempts at prevention of disability among the elderly and in the development of treatment resources.

GROUPS OF ELDERLY ALCOHOLICS

Evidence has been presented that suggests that alcohol abuse among the elderly is a significant problem requiring professional attention, particularly in the area of the provision of treatment services tailored to meet the specific needs of the elderly alcoholic. The question arises as to what these needs may be. Are elderly alcoholics different from younger alcoholics and, if so, in what ways?

It has been suggested that there are at least two distinct groups of elderly alcoholics with differing factors contributing to the development of their drinking problem. Simon and associates,[23] in studying psychiatric admissions of elderly patients, noted that 23 percent were alcoholics. Of this 23 percent, 7 percent became alcoholic after the age of sixty, and 16 percent became alcoholic before age sixty and presumably had long-standing histories of alcohol abuse. This observation indicates that about one third of elderly alcoholics develop a drinking problem in later life, and two-thirds are long-standing alcoholics who manage to drink heavily until old age.

Rosin and Glatt[19] reviewed 103 cases of patients over age sixty-five who were either seen on psychiatric home consultations, were admitted to a regional alcoholism unit, or were admitted to a hospital's geriatric unit. They also found two distinct groups of alcoholics among the patients in their study. About two thirds of the patients in one group were long-standing problem drinkers whose alcoholism persisted as they grew older. This group was noted to have personality factors similar to those found among younger alcoholics. The second group, which represented one third of the patients, developed drinking problems in later life associated with depression, bereavement, retirement, loneliness, marital stress, and physical illness, that is, stresses often associated with aging. The authors noted that there were more women than men in this group of elderly alcoholics, in contrast to the predominance of men among younger alcoholics.

Carruth and his associates[5] reported, however, that their data indicated three distinct types of alcoholics. One type consisted of individuals who had no history of a drinking problem prior to old age and had developed the problem during old age; a second group consisted of individuals who intermittently experienced problems with alcohol but in old age developed a persistent pattern of alcohol abuse; the third group consisted of individuals who had a long history of alcoholism and continued their problem into old age. For practical purposes, however, it would seem that the last two groups are simply alcoholics of long-standing with different manifest patterns of alcohol abuse during their younger years.

Zimberg[27] noted in his work in various health and mental health settings that there are two distinct types of elderly alcoholics and that the ratio of early-onset to late-onset problem drinking is about two to one. However, since there seems to be a natural tendency toward spontaneous remission in many, if not all, long-standing alcoholics as they grow older, the question arises as to why some long-standing alcoholics persist in their self-destructive drinking patterns. It is possible that the stresses of aging not only can lead to the development of late-onset alcoholism but also can contribute to the perpetuation of long-standing alcoholism. An individual with early-onset alcoholism may find that the problems and stresses of old age provide further rationalizations to continue to drink heavily. This possibility leads to the consideration of treatment approaches for elderly alcoholics.

TREATMENT OF ELDERLY ALCOHOLICS

Based on his experience in providing medical and supportive therapy to seven elderly alcoholics in the community, Droller concluded, "The most important therapy is social. These elderly alcoholics (once they are sober and circulation and metabolism have been suitably propped up) respond immediately to the company of their contemporaries and purposeful rehabilitation. This should be arranged as a training program with physiotherapists and occupational therapists."[9]

Rosin and Glatt[19] indicated in their study that environmental manipulation and improvement in the medical condition of the patients were beneficial and resulted in improvement. The day hospital or home visiting by staff or good neighbors were services that were most beneficial.

Zimberg[27] reported from his experience with elderly alcoholics in a nursing home environment, a medical home care program, and a geriatric psychiatric outpatient program that both types of elderly alcoholics (late- and early-onset) were responsive to therapeutic intervention in relation to their alcoholism. Depression, social isolation, and feelings of hopelessness were common in both groups. When these patients were involved in group discussions with other elderly individuals (who did not have drinking problems) and were provided with antidepressant medications and social and recreational activities, they responded by discontinuation of their drinking. It seems that as the aging-related stress factors in these people were reduced, they gave up alcohol with little difficulty and, therefore, seemed to have a better prognosis for recovery than younger alcoholics.

It seems likely that services can best be provided in programs serving the elderly rather than in alcoholism programs. Specialized programs dealing with the elderly alcohol abuser, staffed by personnel knowledgeable about alcoholism and the psychosocial aspects of aging, can establish specialized services for the elderly alcoholics within programs for the elderly, such as senior centers or nursing homes. They can also be developed by establishing liaison relationships with existing alcoholism programs by using consultants expert in the treatment of alcoholism working together with staff of the aging service program.

PREVENTION OF ALCOHOLISM AMONG THE ELDERLY

Rosin and Glatt[19] have documented that stress factors such as loss of loved ones, retirement, loneliness, physical illness, and marital stress were environmental factors that contributed to alcohol abuse among the elderly. They also suggested that ". . . manipulation of the environment and improvement in the medical condition are often beneficial. . . . Preretirement courses help to avoid a social vacuum after the person leaves work. Transfer to a welfare home can be a timely preventive of further social and alcoholic deterioration in some cases."

Many of the stresses of aging can be reduced or eliminated through the development of an effective network of services for the elderly involving social services, economic and housing assistance, physical health care, and psychological counseling. Although the development of senile dementia and other chronic brain syndromes cannot be reversed at the present stage of medical knowledge, the impact of such disorders and their effect on functional capacity can be reduced by effective and comprehensive services.[25] If alcohol abuse develops in the elderly as a reaction to such problems or, in the case of long-standing alcoholics does not spontaneously remit, reducing the impact of senile dementia may help to reduce alcoholism among the elderly.

It has been proposed that the well-known sociability effects of alcohol might be helpful for elderly individuals experiencing behavioral and mood problems. Becker and Cesar[2] investigated the use of beer on a group of elderly psychiatric patients in a mental hospital compared to a similar group given fruit juice. After eleven weeks they noted increased social interaction in the group given beer but no improvement in ward behavior outside these group sessions for either group. Chien, Stotsky, and Cole[6] reported positive results from the use of alcohol in a nursing home to improve ward sociability and manageability of patients: "Following a four-week control period, 64 nursing home patients receiving doxepin, other psychoactive drugs, or no medication were placed on an alcohol regimen of beer or wine in the ward or in a simulated pub set-up. The alcohol produced significant improvement in all groups, especially the doxepin group. However, the pub milieu did not demonstrate a significant superiority over ward milieu."

The results in these two studies should be expected, since the sociability effects of alcohol are well known. It should be noted, however, that the two studies reported above studied the effects of alcohol on behavior for only eleven and four weeks, respectively, much too short a time to determine any possible detrimental effects which might ensue through the continued use of alcohol. Alcohol is a potentially addicting substance, and, since older people are more susceptible to sedative-hypnotic drugs, it may be that tolerance to alcohol develops more rapidly in an elderly person. With the continued use of alcohol, more might be required to produce the same euphoriant effects. Patients developing tolerance may ask for more beer and wine and may be denied it by the staff, which may create serious management problems. Nursing homes in particular may be prone to this problem, and, since there is evidence that more and more alcoholic patients are being placed in nursing homes,[13] a widespread practice of using alcohol within an institutional setting may result in iatrogenic alcoholism.

The use of alcohol as a beverage may have some value when used outside the institutional setting during picnics and outings as part of normal social and recreational activities operated as part of a therapeutic community program for institutionalized elderly. However, the principles of the therapeutic community approach in which elderly patients participate with staff in meaningful activities fostering self-help and concern for other patients can produce far more significant changes in behavior and functional capacities than alcohol. It is easy to give a drug, including alcohol, in an effort to improve mood and behavior. In fact, many physicians often prescribe alcohol for elderly patients who have experienced loss of appetite or insomnia, when often such symptoms are manifestations of depression. However, there are far more effective antidepressant drugs than alcohol, and sociability can better be fostered through effective staff-patient and patient-patient interactions without the danger of possibly producing iatrogenic alcoholism.[3] It is important for physicians to become more aware of social, physical, and psychological stresses of aging and to be able to recognize depression in an elderly person. Current psychosocial therapies, skillfully applied, can treat the elderly more effectively than through any palliative effects of alcohol.

Another major problem in dealing with alcoholism in general has been the unwillingness of physicians to recognize the problem and make a diagnosis and their general feeling of hopelessness about treating alcoholics; these problems are even more severe in relation to elderly patients.[14, 24]

It is necessary for physicians and other health care professionals to become knowledgeable concerning alcohol and alcoholism and its use in the United States. With such knowledge, they will be better able to diagnose individuals with alcoholism early in their course, refer them for appropriate treatment, and avoid the tendency to use alcohol as a therapeutic agent.

REFERENCES

1. Bailey, M. B., Haberman, P. W., and Alksne, H.: The epidemiology of alcoholism in an urban residential area. *Q J Stud Alcohol*, 26:19-40, 1965.
2. Becker, P. W. and Cesar, J. A.: Use of beer in geriatric psychiatric patient groups. *Psychol Rep*, 33:182, 1973.
3. Blume, S. B.: Iatrogenic alcoholism. *Q J Stud Alcohol*, 34:1348-1352, 1973.
4. Cahalan, D., Cisin, I. H., and Crossley, H. M.: *American Drinking Practices: A National Study of Drinking Behavior and Attitudes*. New Brunswick, New Jersey, Rutgers Center of Alcohol Studies, 1969.
5. Carruth, B., Williams, E. P., Mysak, P., and Boudreaux, L.: *Community Care Providers and the Older Problem Drinker*. Paper presented

to the General Sessions of the Alcohol and Drug Problems Association of North America, Sept. 23-28, 1973.
6. Chien, C., Stotsky, B. A., and Cole, J. O.: Psychiatric treatment for nursing home patients: Drug, alcohol and milieu. *Am J Psychiatry, 130*:543-548, 1973.
7. deLint, J.: The prevention of alcoholism. *Prev Med, 3*:24-35, 1974.
8. Drew, L. R. H.: Alcoholism as a self-limiting disease. *Q J Stud Alcohol, 29*:956-967, 1968.
9. Droller, H.: Some aspects of alcoholism in the elderly. *Lancet, 2*:137-139, 1964.
10. Epstein, L. J., Mills, C., and Simon, A.: Antisocial behavior of the elderly. *Compr Psychiatry, 11*:36-42, 1970.
11. Faris, D.: The prevention of alcoholism and economic alcoholism. *Prev Med, 3*:36-48, 1974.
12. Gorwitz, K., Bahn, A., Warthen, F. J., and Cooper, M.: Some epidemiological data on alcoholism in Maryland. *Q J Stud Alcohol, 31*:423-443, 1970.
13. Linn, M. W., Linn, B. S., and Greenwald, S. R.: The alcoholic patient in the nursing home. *Aging Hum Dev, 3*:273-277, 1972.
14. Lisansky, E. T.: Why physicians avoid early diagnosis of alcoholism. *NY State J Med, 75*:1788-1792, 1975.
15. Locke, B. Z., Kramer, M., and Pasamanick, B.: Alcoholic psychoses among first admissions to public mental health hospitals in Ohio. *Q J Stud Alcohol, 21*:457-474, 1960.
16. Malzberg, B.: A study of first admissions with alcoholic psychoses in New York State, 1943-1944. *Q J Stud Alcohol, 8*:274-295, 1947.
17. McCusker, J., Cherubin, C. E., and Zimberg, S.: Prevalence of alcoholism in general municipal hospital population. *NY State J Med, 71*:751-754, 1971.
18. National Institute on Alcohol Abuse and Alcoholism: *Alcohol and Health.* Washington, D.C., U.S. Govt Print Office, 1971.
19. Rosin, A. J. and Glatt, M. M.: Alcohol excess in the elderly. *Q J Stud Alcohol, 32*:52-59, 1971.
20. Schmidt, W. and deLint, J.: Causes of death of alcoholics. *Q J Stud Alcohol, 33*:171-185, 1972.
21. Schuckit, M. A. and Miller, P. L.: *Alcoholism in Elderly Men: A Survey of a General Medical Ward.* Paper presented to the Sixth Annual Medical-Scientific Session of the National Alcoholism Forum, Milwaukee, Wisconsin, Apr. 28-29, 1975.
22. Siassi, I., Crocetti, G., and Spiro, H. R.: Drinking patterns and alcoholism in a blue collar population. *Q J Stud Alcohol, 34*:917-926, 1973.
23. Simon, A., Epstein, L. J., and Reynolds, L.: Alcoholism in the geriatric mentally ill. *Geriatrics, 23*:125-131, 1968.

24. Straus, R.: Medical practice and the alcoholic. *Ann Am Acad Pol Soc Sci, 315*:117-124, 1958.
25. Zimberg, S.: Outpatient geriatric psychiatry in an urban ghetto with nonprofessional workers. *Am J Psychiatry, 125*:1697-1702, 1969.
26. ———: The psychiatrist and medical home care: Geriatric psychiatry in the Harlem community. *Am J Psychiatry, 127*:1062-1066, 1971.
27. ———: The elderly alcoholic. *Gerontologist, 14*:221-224, 1974.

Chapter 4

ACUTE DRUG REACTIONS AMONG THE ELDERLY*

DAVID M. PETERSEN, PH.D.
CHARLES W. THOMAS, PH.D.

DRUG USE AND MISUSE among the elderly continues to be a neglected area of research in the field of social gerontology. Standard textbooks, for example, devote little or no attention to the topic.[1, 8, 10, 13, 14] Further, despite the rapid growth of literature on other drug-related issues, few research projects have focused upon drug use patterns among the elderly.[2-4] Social gerontologists are apparently preoccupied with other matters.† This chapter is concerned with one of the most crucial and vexing aspects of the drug problem in the United States, a problem of considerable importance to those concerned with the problems of the aged: the acute drug reaction (overdose). Specifically, this paper provides basic source data on elderly persons who were treated for nonfatal but acute drug reactions in a hospital emergency room and, in particular, the paper both describes the demographic and social characteristics of these patients and provides comparisons of this elderly cohort with all acute drug reaction admissions.

---

* From "Acute Drug Reactions Among the Elderly," *Journal of Gerontology*, 30 (Sept., 1975):552-556. Reprinted by permission.

† A considerable body of literature dealing with the aged and drugs has arisen in recent years, however, as health professionals have directed their attention to the effect of the aging process on pharmacological efficacy and safety. Interest has centered upon pharmacological issues such as drug side effects, drug interactions, and drug-related disorders, as well as clinical issues including long-term drug management and drug management of the psychiatrically ill.[6, 7] In addition, information on expenditures for health services and supplies, types of drugs commonly prescribed, number and costs of prescriptions for the elderly has been researched by the Task Force on Prescription Drugs.[12]

Data for the present study were gathered from the patient records of 1,128 persons treated for an acute drug reaction at Jackson Memorial Hospital, Miami, Dade County, Florida, during 1972. For the purposes of this study, an acute drug reaction was defined as those effects resulting from drug ingestion that either produced interference with adequate social functioning or that were subjectively perceived as so unpleasant that the user sought assistance in the hospital emergency room.[11] Excluded from our analysis are 117 subjects admitted to the emergency room for other such drug-related reasons as hepatitis, poisonings, and addiction detoxification. In the main, evidence regarding documentation of the overdose situation was based upon a medical history gathered from the patient or some accompanying person by the attending staff in the emergency room. In some cases, verification of drug abuse diagnosis was derived from laboratory analysis.

GENERAL CHARACTERISTICS OF SIXTY AGED ADMISSIONS FOR ACUTE DRUG REACTIONS

Previous research has indicated that admissions to Jackson Memorial Hospital, Miami, Florida, for emergency treatment of drug overdoses occur preponderantly among the young.[5, 9] The age-category under examination here, those aged fifty and over (senior adulthood), accounts for only 5.4 percent of all admissions to this southern Florida emergency room. The age-range for these admissions was from fifty to eighty years. The mean age for this cohort was 59.6 years, as contrasted to 27.6 years for all overdose admissions during 1972 (N=1,128).

A distribution by sex (Table 4-I) for the sixty drug overdoses shows that aged admissions were more likely to be females than males (68.4% vs. 31.6%). In addition, a comparison of the aged cohort with all admissions reveals a greater concentration of females among the aged group as well (68.4% vs. 58.6%). Acute drug overdose admissions also varied according to the race of these substance abusers; 85 percent of these aged patients were white (Table 4-I). When the aged cohort is compared with all admissions, it is found that black patients account for only 15 percent of the aged admissions but 33 percent of the total admissions for 1972. Although white females were far more likely to be admitted for an acute overdose reaction than any other race-sex grouping for both the aged cohort and all admissions, the proportion is much more striking among the aged (61.7% vs. 38.4%). Indeed, white females account for almost two-thirds of all admissions among the aged.

In order to contrast the aforementioned data with the general population characteristics of the area serviced by the hospital, race, sex, and age comparisons were made with the most recent census data on Dade County, Florida. As indicated in Table 4-II, persons over age fifty are not overrepresented among emergency room admissions for acute drug reactions.

As indicated in Table 4-III, female admissions exceed their distribution for Dade County as a whole (68.4% vs. 55.3%), as do white female admissions (61.7% vs. 51.4%). Similarly, black

TABLE 4-I

CHARACTERISTICS OF SIXTY AGED PATIENTS COMPARED TO ALL PATIENTS ADMITTED FOR EMERGENCY TREATMENT OF ACUTE DRUG REACTIONS, JACKSON MEMORIAL HOSPITAL, MIAMI, FLORIDA (1972)

		Aged Admissions (N = 60) N	%	Total Admissions (N = 1,128) N	%
A.	Race-Sex Distribution				
	White male	14	23.3	322	28.6
	White female	37	61.7	433	38.4
	Black male	5	8.3	144	12.8
	Black female	4	6.7	228	20.2
		60	100.0	1,127	100.0
B.	Number of Substances Abused (excluding alcohol)				
	Single-substance use	32	68.1	720	76.5
	Multiple-substance use	15	31.9	221	23.5
		47	100.0	941	100.0
C.	Alcohol-Drug Use in Combination				
	Present	5	8.3	123	10.9
	Not present	55	91.7	1,005	89.1
		60	100.0	1,128	100.0
D.	Suicide Attempt				
	Yes	14	35.0	272	33.7
	No	26	65.0	535	66.3
		40	100.0	807	100.0

Note: Columns in all tables may not exactly equal 100.0 due to rounding error.

TABLE 4-II

AGE DISTRIBUTION FOR DADE COUNTY, FLORIDA, COMPARED TO ALL ACUTE DRUG REACTION ADMISSIONS TO THE DADE COUNTY HOSPITAL EMERGENCY ROOM, JACKSON MEMORIAL HOSPITAL, MIAMI, FLORIDA (1972)

Age Distribution* (Years of Age)	Total Population of Dade County (1970) %	Total Admissions to Emergency Room (1972) %
14-17	8.8	15.5
18-24	13.0	42.0
25-34	14.9	21.7
35-49	24.3	15.4
50 and over	39.0	5.4

* Since no persons under the age of fourteen sought treatment for an acute drug reaction at the emergency room, persons under the age of fourteen in Dade County were omitted from this analysis.

TABLE 4-III

RACE AND SEX DISTRIBUTION FOR PERSONS OVER FIFTY FOR DADE COUNTY, FLORIDA, COMPARED TO THE SIXTY AGED ACUTE DRUG REACTION ADMISSIONS TO THE DADE COUNTY HOSPITAL EMERGENCY ROOM, JACKSON MEMORIAL HOSPITAL, MIAMI, FLORIDA (1972)

Race-Sex Distribution	Population Over 50 for Dade County (1970) %	Aged Admissions to Emergency Room (1972) %
White males	41.4	23.3
White females	51.4	61.7
Black males	3.3	8.3
Black females	3.9	6.7
Total whites	92.8	85.0
Total blacks	7.2	15.0
Total males	44.7	31.6
Total females	55.3	68.4

admissions to the hospital emergency room exceed their distribution in Dade County by more than two to one (15.0% vs. 7.2%). Black male admissions to the hospital exceed their distribution in the hospital service area (8.3% vs. 3.3%) by a slightly greater margin than black female admissions (6.7% vs. 3.9%).

In examining the number of substances used (excluding alcohol) prior to their admission to the hospital emergency room, it was found the majority of these patients listed only one substance as being responsible for their overdose admission (*see* Table 4-I). Still, in almost one-fourth of all admissions (23.5%), the patient admitted that two or more substances had been used together. The proportion of multiple-substance use prior to an acute drug reaction is even higher among the aged patients (31.9%). In addition, alcohol use in combination with other substance abuse was present in 8.3 percent of the aged cohort admissions and in 10.9 percent of the total admissions. Thus, the aged admissions are somewhat more likely to report multiple-substance abuse but slightly less likely to have also used alcohol immediately prior to their acute reaction.

The reasons advanced for drug use include the desire for a euphoric effect, self-medication, and so on. These types of "accidental" overdoses account for the majority of the admissions for both the total admissions and the aged cohort (*see* Table 4-I). At the same time, however, in one-third of these cases, the acute drug reactions were associated with suicide attempts. Little difference exists between the aged admissions and the total admissions on this dimension (35.0% and 33.7%, respectively).

PRIMARY SUBSTANCE OF ABUSE ASSOCIATED WITH ADMISSION FOR TREATMENT

Each patient admitted for the treatment of an acute drug reaction was classified according to the primary substance responsible for the admission. Of those patients who had abused two or more substances, designation of the main substance was determined on a case-to-case basis, according to the amount of each substance ingested and/or whether the substance(s) could be identified as having a legitimate medical usage. Information of substance use prior to admission was unknown for 195 (17.3%) of the total admissions and for 13 (21.7%) of the aged admissions.

A wide variety of substances were identified as having caused the acute drug reactions; 30 different drugs were identified by the aged admissions and some 125 by the total admissions. Of particular significance is the fact that the majority of all admissions were for the misuse of drugs that had been both legally manufactured and distributed. More than three-fourths of the total admissions in 1972 (79.4%) were identified as resulting from substances legally available by either prescription or over-the-

TABLE 4-IV

PRIMARY SUBSTANCE OF ABUSE FOR FORTY-SEVEN AGED PATIENTS COMPARED TO ALL PATIENTS ADMITTED FOR EMERGENCY TREATMENT OF ACUTE DRUG REACTIONS, JACKSON MEMORIAL HOSPITAL, MIAMI, FLORIDA (1972)

		Aged Admissions (N = 47)		Total Admissions (N = 933)	
		N	%	N	%
A.	Illicit substances				
	Heroin	—	—	83	8.9
	Hallucinogens (LSD)	—	—	82	8.8
	Inhalants (glue)	—	—	15	1.6
	Stimulants (cocaine)	—	—	12	1.3
	Subtotal	—	—	192	20.6
B.	Legal substances				
	Methadone	1	2.1	12	1.3
	Narcotics (Demerol)	—	—	13	1.4
	Non-narcotic analgesics (Darvon)	5	10.6	94	10.1
	Tranquilizers (Librium)	15	31.9	228	24.4
	Sedatives (Seconal)	23	49.0	335	35.9
	Stimulants (Dexedrine)	—	—	19	2.0
	Other (quinine, atropine)	3	6.4	40	4.3
	Subtotal	47	100.0	741	79.4
	Total	47	100.0	933	100.0

counter without prescription. All admissions among the aged cohort resulted from legally available drugs (Table 4-IV). (There is no means of determining from the medical histories, however, by which means these patients acquired these drugs.) Stated differently, *there were no admissions among those patients fifty and over that were the result of ingestion of an illicit substance.* Moreover, 80.9 percent of acute drug reactions among the elderly involve the misuse or abuse of a legal psychotropic drug (sedatives and tranquilizers), and comparable data for the total number of admissions indicate 60.3 percent of all acute reactions involve the psychotropic drugs. Overdoses from non-narcotic analgesics account for an additional 10.6 percent of the aged admissions. Thus, nine of every ten drugs resulting in an acute reaction among the elderly are either a sedative, tranquilizer, or non-narcotic analgesic. Specifically, the most frequently misused drugs, ranked according to frequency of abuse, are diazepam (Valium), a tranquilizer; sodium secobarbital and sodium amobarbital (Tuinal), a hypnotic; phenobarbital, a sedative; and propoxyphene hydrochloride (Darvon), a non-narcotic analgesic. Further analysis of the relationship between type of substance and the race and sex of the aged overdose patients indicates that the use of tranquilizers, sedatives, and non-narcotic analgesics prior to the acute drug reaction experience is most consistent for whites and females. (Tabular material is available from the authors.)

DISCUSSION

Consumption rates of drugs in the United States suggest that the elderly are exposed to many more drugs of potential abuse than other age-groups. Data for the prescription drugs alone reveal that those over sixty-five years, while comprising roughly one-tenth of the population, received one-fourth of all prescriptions written in 1967. One can assume that they also consume an equally substantial proportion of over-the-counter drugs. The three most prescribed drugs for the elderly include two tranquilizers, Valium and Librium, and a non-narcotic analgesic, Darvon.[12]

The data from the present study are quite conclusive in documenting the dangers of the misuse of the psychotropics (sedatives and minor tranquilizers) among the elderly. The significance of these drugs as causal agents in the majority of accidental overdose and suicidal gesturing cases cannot be denied. Although further data collection and analysis is required for confirmation, our observations suggest that chronic misuse (increased dosage and/or increased frequency of consumption) resulting in accidental overdose is greater with minor tranquilizers than with sedatives, but deliberate overdoses more frequently involve sedatives. Regardless of such future determinations, emergency room personnel *must* be made aware of the fact that the overwhelming majority of all acute drug reactions among the elderly involve the life-threatening problems caused by an overdose of sedatives or tranquilizers.

Although acute drug reactions resulting from the abuse or misuse of drugs are widely recognized occurrences among drug users, medical practitioners, and researchers, there has been a surprisingly meager amount of cumulative scientific insight into the problem. There are a number of reasons for this state of affairs, including the fact that existing studies in the area have serious problems in research design and sampling. Most research has used clinical samples of patients who are already suffering from some problem concurrent with or related to drug usage. This problem is made more serious because these studies do not have control groups of drug users who have not had acute drug reactions, thus making it difficult to unravel existing problems, such as psychiatric problems and adverse reactions to drug experiences. Our research suffers from similar limitations in that only data from those individuals who sought assistance for their adverse drug reaction in a hospital emergency room setting is available. We do not, then, have any information regarding those persons who managed their overdose experience without seeking outside assistance. For this reason, we cannot presume that those individuals who reach a hospital are identical to those who manage their problem in the community, and this is an important area for future research. Our findings suggest, however, that the predominance of drug problems among men in the younger ages appears to recede in later years and that there is a greater likelihood of encountering such acute drug problems as overdosing among elderly women rather than among men.

Because the occurrence of acute drug reactions is related to both the number and frequency of drug exposures, we surmise from the drug-use behavior of the elderly that they are quite prone to become victims of overdosing. Our analysis of emergency room admissions, however, suggests that many overdoses and other adverse reactions to drugs among the elderly are not being managed in a hospital setting.

SUMMARY

The acute drug reaction is just one of a variety of forms of drug abuse among the elderly that is of major significance but that has received little or no attention. While the good that drugs can do within the limits of a medically supervised regimen is recognized, it may not be generally recognized that, by virtue of the natural aging process, the elderly are more likely to be receiving a variety of drugs because of the increased rate of physical illness, psychiatric disorders, and such common geriatric problems as loneliness, boredom, and depression. The present study has provided evidence regarding one aspect of the serious overuse of drugs by elderly Americans.

Some of the striking features regarding hospital emergency room admissions for acute drug reactions among the elderly may be concisely summarized:

1. Acute drug reaction cases among the admissions we examined were more likely to be females than males (58.6% vs. 41.4%). This imbalance is even stronger when aged female admissions are compared with their male counterparts (68.4% vs. 31.6%).

2. The vast majority of acute drug reactions involve whites (85.0%). Further, white females were more likely to be admitted for treatment of an acute reaction than any other race-sex cohort, accounting for almost two-thirds (61.7%) of all admissions among the aged.

3. In terms of proportional representation, the aged are not overrepresented among all admissions for acute overdose reactions when comparisons are made with census data for the general population serviced by the hospital (Dade County, Florida). When race and sex data are examined, however, white females and blacks of both sexes are found to be overrepresented among the aged admissions.

4. In almost one-third of the cases (31.9%), the aged patients had mixed two or more substances together prior to their adverse drug reaction (contrasted to 23.5% among all admissions). In addition, alcohol use in combination with other substance use was present in 8.3 percent of the aged admissions (contrasted to 10.9% among all admissions).

5. Some one-third of both the aged admissions and the total admissions admit they were consciously trying to commit suicide (35.0% and 33.7%, respectively).

6. Although there are narcotic users among the elderly, the greater problem involves prescription drugs. No aged patient was admitted during the study period as the result of ingestion of an illicit substance. Almost one-fourth (20.6%) of the total admissions, however, were the result of abuse of an illicit substance, e.g. heroin or hallucinogens.

7. Slightly over 80 percent (80.9%) of all acute drug reactions among the elderly involve the misuse or abuse of a legally manufactured and distributed psychotropic (sedatives and tran-

quilizers). Overdoses from non-narcotic analgesics account for an additional 10.6 percent of the aged admissions.

8. The most frequently misused drugs among the aged include Valium, Tuinal, phenobarbital, and Darvon.

REFERENCES

1. Atchley, R. C.: *The Social Forces in Later Life: An Introduction to Social Gerontology.* Belmont, California, Wadsworth Pub, 1972.
2. Barton, R. and Hurst, L.: Unnecessary use of tranquilizers in elderly patients. *Br J Psychiatry, 112*:989-990, 1966.
3. Capel, W. C. and Stewart, G. T.: The management of drug abuse in aging populations: New Orleans findings. *J Drug Issues, 1*:114-120, 1971.
4. Capel, W. C., Goldsmith, B. M., Waddell, K. J., and Stewart, G. T.: The aging narcotic addict: An increasing problem for the next decades. *J Gerontol, 27*:102-106, 1972.
5. Chambers, C. D., Petersen, D. M., and Newman, S. C.: The acute drug reaction in a hospital emergency room: A demographic and social assessment. *J Fla Med Assoc, 62*:40-42, 1975.
6. Davis, R. H. and Smith, W. K. (Eds.): *Drugs and the Elderly.* Los Angeles, Ethel Percy Andrus Gerontology Center, U of S Cal, 1973.
7. Fann, W. E. and Maddox, G. L. (Eds.): *Drug Issues in Geropsychiatry.* Baltimore, Williams & Wilkins, 1974.
8. Koller, M. R.: *Social Gerontology.* New York, Random House, 1968.
9. Petersen, D. M. and Chambers, C. D.: Demographic characteristics of emergency room admissions for acute drug reactions. *Int J Addict, 10*:963-975, 1975.
10. Riley, M. W. and Foner, A.: *Aging and Society.* New York, Russell Sage, 1968.
11. Smith, D. E. and Mehl, C.: An analysis of marijuana toxicity. In D. E. Smith (Ed.): *The New Social Drug.* Englewood Cliffs, New Jersey, Prentice-Hall, 1970.
12. Task Force on Prescription Drugs: *The Drug Users.* Washington, D.C., U.S. Govt Print Office, 1968.
13. Tibbitts, C. (Ed.): *Handbook of Social Gerontology: Societal Aspects of Aging.* Chicago, U of Chicago Pr, 1960.
14. Vedder, C. B. (Ed.): *Gerontology: A Book of Readings.* Springfield, Thomas, 1963.

Section II

PHARMACOLOGY, PHARMACY, AND
THE ELDERLY PATIENT

Chapter 5

SIDE EFFECTS OF DRUGS IN THE ELDERLY

RONALD J. ZIANCE, PH.D.

THIS CHAPTER NEGLECTS the impressive benefits attributed to the judicious use of drugs in humans but instead focuses on the undesirable and, at times, serious side effects produced by several categories of drugs routinely consumed by the geriatric population. The greater incidence of adverse side effects in the elderly can be partially attributed to several age-related physiological alterations that may influence the life cycle of the drug, host sensitivity, and thus the effects of various drugs in the elderly.

The absorption of an oral medication from the gastrointestinal tract into blood vessels depends upon drug dispersion and solubility of the drug in the intestines.[10] Drug absorption from the stomach[58,115] and intestines depends upon the acidic or alkaline environment within these organs; thus, the fact that older persons have a reduced output of gastric acid[6] strongly suggests that the absorption of some drugs differs in the elderly versus the young drug recipient. Many drugs are transported across biological membranes via passive or active transport processes.[116] Both of these transport processes are significantly reduced in the elderly, which may be a reflection of the reduced number of intestinal absorbing cells coincident with the aging process.[10] Such effects also reduce drug absorption from the gastrointestinal tract. The action of most drugs is terminated by metabolism via liver enzymes and subsequent elimination by the kidneys.[135] Typically, the liver of an older person has a decreased capacity to metabolize drugs to an inactive form prior to elimination by the kidneys.[51] In normal men over forty years of age, there is a correlation between age and declining kidney function, as evidenced by the fact that anatomic narrowing of blood vessels and a decreased cardiac output result in a 50 percent decrease of renal plasma blood flow between the ages of twenty and ninety.[12, 40, 55] It is not uncommon for the rate of urine formation in the elderly to be one-third less that of a younger population.[93, 130] It is not expected that all drugs fit into the same absorption-elimination scheme nor be uniformly influenced by the age-related defects mentioned above. Thus, upon oral ingestion and adequate absorption of a drug from the stomach or intestine, impaired liver and kidney function result in high blood concentration of the drug if the main route of drug elimination is liver metabolism followed by urinary excretion.[3, 113] Such information indicates that the normal adult dose of such a drug should be reduced if given to an elderly individual. The same advice also applies to a drug that is not normally metabolized by the liver and reaches the age-compromised kidney in an unchanged state, since the increased content of the drug in blood predisposes the patient to its toxic effects.[31] Accordingly, many physicians consider it good practice to prescribe doses of medication one-half to one-third the normal adult dosage to geriatric patients.[53]

In contrast, if an orally administered drug undergoes reduced absorption into the blood followed by normal rates of metabolism and elimination, it may be necessary to increase the dosage so that adequate blood levels of the drug are achieved to render the desired therapeutic response.

On the basis of the many possible patterns of absorption, metabolism, and elimination of drugs, it is not surprising that elderly patients undergo a greater incidence of side effects from prescription drugs. In this regard, it is also imperative not to overlook the sizeable voluntary consumption of nonprescription drugs by the elderly.

Age modifications of drug activity appear to be most common to drugs that act on the central nervous system (CNS).[9] By the seventh decade, the weight of the human brain decreases by about 7 percent.[57] In some regions of the human brain, more than 20 percent of the neurons may be lost by the age of seventy,[15] with the greatest decrease of neuronal population occurring in the cerebral cortex.[11] The decreased oxygen consumption by the aged brain is thought to be due to the decreased number of functional neurons.[53, 59] There seems to be general agreement that many of the behavioral and physiological manifestations of aging are associated with the progressive loss of brain neurons.[65] It is thought that alterations in the mental behavior of older patients may induce abnormal psychologic responses to various drugs,[65] especially those drugs which excite or depress the CNS. As a general rule, CNS depressants have an increased potency, whereas CNS stimulants exert a reduced activity in the aged brain.[9, 38]

The unusual effects of many centrally acting drugs have been explained in the following manner. The normal interaction and balance among the various brain regions is altered by the aging process, since the rate of neuron loss varies in different regions of the brain. The end result is deterioration of integrated brain function, which is expressed as an altered reactivity and sensitivity of the aged brain to centrally acting drugs.[65] Thus, the administration of certain drugs that are relatively innocuous to younger individuals may produce dangerous reactions in the elderly.[82] Drugs acting on both the central and peripheral nervous systems generally show significant changes in their central effects, but their peripheral effects remain unchanged.[38] Thus, the sedative phenobarbital may cause confusion, excitement, and agitation in the elderly patient to such an extent that the careful physician often avoids its use in geriatric patients.[41, 43]

The following information provides some insight into the problems at hand. Hurwitz and Wade reported that the rate of adverse drug effects of patients over seventy years of age was twice that of patients sixty to sixty-nine years old.[64] It is interesting to note that the study was performed in a hospital and that the drugs were administered by the nursing personnel. The problem may be further compounded if elderly patients are relied upon to take the correct doses of prescribed drugs at home. The elderly patient is often directed to consume several different medications each day, since more than one disease state is usually being treated.[132] Medication errors by the elderly patient may be attributable to a poor memory, depression, or a resistant attitude toward drugs.[71] Thus, it is not surprising that 60 percent of chronically ill elderly persons who administered their own medications at home made errors, such as dose omission, inaccurate dosage, or improper timing or sequence of medication.[119]

Of equal importance is the fact that the incidence of severe adverse effects is considerably increased following the use of multiple drugs by the elderly.[81, 104] During a three-year period, 2.9 percent of 6,063 admissions of all ages to a Florida medical service, excluding suicide attempts and drug abuse, were due to drug-induced illnesses. Notably, proportionately more patients between the ages of sixty and eighty years of age were admitted because of drug reactions.[19]

It is imperative that directions for drugs taken by the elderly at home be as simple as possible and that the dosage regimen fit into the patient's daily routine.[119] It is generally accepted that many adverse drug reactions in the elderly are not reported and are thus untreated, because members of the subject's family may misinterpret a drug side effect as just another inevitable sign of progressing old age.[23, 120]

It is appropriate to consider in greater detail the adverse effects produced by several categories of drugs routinely consumed by the elderly. The following discussion indicates the main pharmacologic category of the drugs considered plus the generic and, in parentheses, trade name(s) of representative products available in the United States. Although it is impossible to adequately consider each of the many drug categories or every drug within a category which causes adverse effects in the elderly, this discussion of several selected drugs serves as an index to the magnitude of the problem.

CNS-ACTING DRUGS

In a typical year in the United States, 370 million prescriptions are dispensed for drugs whose main action is to either depress or stimulate the CNS. Drug consumption is one activity that is not compromised by old age, since the geriatric population is probably a larger consumer of CNS-acting drugs than any other population group.[81]

Anti-Parkinson Drugs

L-dopa, L-3,4-dihydroxyphenylalanine (Dopar®, Larodopa®): Parkinson's disease, which afflicts 1.8 of every 1,000 subjects of all ages and 7 of every 1,000 subjects over fifty years of age,[78, 134] is an insidious abnormality produced by degeneration of certain nerves of the brain that normally release the chemical dopamine. This deficit of brain dopamine results in symptoms of tremors and rigidity of skeletal muscle and/or akinesia[37, 62] (slowness of and difficulty in initiation of body movements). L-dopa, which is converted to dopamine within the brain, is considered to be the single most effective drug for controlling Parkinson's disease.[87] The symptoms are alleviated in approximately two-thirds of recipient patients.[70, 79] Some clinical studies report that skeletal muscle rigidity is improved more than tremor;[45, 87] however, the reverse has also been reported.[106] The dosage of L-dopa must be individualized for each patient, since after several months of therapy some patients may experience tolerance (decreased therapeutic effect) to L-dopa therapy, which requires alteration of dosage. The age of the patient at the time of therapy initiation is important, since younger patients exhibit a more satisfactory overall response than older patients.[45, 94]

L-dopa therapy is certainly not devoid of disturbing side effects, some of which include dyskinesia (characterized by involuntary movements of the limbs); nausea; vomiting; abnormal heart beat; hypotension (low blood pressure); and psychiatric disorders, such as visual hallucinations, disorientation, depression, nightmares, and paranoid ideation.[78, 87, 106] The incidence of these side effects in elderly patients may be appreciated by the report that each of one hundred patients (with a mean age of 60.2 years) experienced at least one adverse reaction to L-dopa therapy.[87]

Several attempts have been made to find a drug that will decrease the incidence of L-dopa side effects. Miller and Nieburg have reported that eight of nine elderly L-dopa recipients who were also treated with L-tryptophan, 1 to 2.5 g daily for two weeks, experienced a clearing of L-dopa-induced psychiatric symptoms and remained free of side effects over an eight-month period.[92] Dyskinesia, the incidence of which has been reported to be as high as 60 percent,[139] is considered to be the most important factor favoring limitation of the chronic use of L-dopa therapy.[72] The L-dopa-induced dyskinetic effects are nonuniform and include involuntary movements of various neck and facial muscles, grimacing, yawning, gnawing, and involuntary movements of the tongue and extremities.[73] Miller also found that L-dopa-induced dyskinesia was completely eliminated in eight of eleven elderly patients who were also treated with daily doses of deanol.[91] Although these results are rather preliminary, these or similar agents may eventually prove to be reliable adjuncts to L-dopa therapy.

Antipsychotic Drugs

Phenothiazines

Chlorpromazine (Thorazine), prochlorperazine (Compazine®), thioridazine (Mellaril), trifluoperazine (Stelazine®), perphenazine (Trilafon®), butaperazine (Repoise®): These drugs belong to a class of compounds known as the *phenothiazines,* the members of which exhibit differences in their antipsychotic potency and propensity to produce certain side effects. The widest application of the phenothiazines is in the treatment of schizophrenia, anxiety, agitation, agitated depression, acute confusional states, alcoholism, and nausea.[26, 53] In the younger age-range, there are some indications that massive doses of phenothiazines may help some patients.[28] However, massive doses of phenothiazines are thought to be no more beneficial than smaller doses in the elderly,[103] although Daniel emphasizes the importance of not using too small a dose in phenothiazine therapy when a large dose is essential.[26] Although there are no age-related differences in the absorption, distribution, metabolism, or excretion of phenothiazines in humans, the aging process results in an increased sensitivity to the therapeutic and toxic effects of the phenothiazines.[53] The elderly are more likely to experience the following phenothiazine-induced side effects, which are generally proportional to dose:[53] mood depression, excessive sedation, toxic confusional reactions, hypotension, fainting, blood disorders, sensitivity to light, Parkinson-like symptoms, and dyskinesia. Approximately 50 percent of geriatric patients who take chlorpromazine experience Parkinson-like symptoms[47, 123] and dyskinesia.[53] The Parkinson reactions are reversible upon reduction or cessation of therapy; however, dyskinesia, which occurs more often in the elderly, may remain for years after discontinuation of therapy.[4, 25, 75] Akathisia (inability to sit still), a predominant phenothiazine side effect in elderly women, has been misdiagnosed as Huntington's chorea[117] and has also been mistaken for increased agitation, with resultant increase in the dosage of the offending drug, which leads to an exacerbation of adverse side effects.[53, 132]

The most common and perhaps the most dangerous side effect of the phenothiazines in the elderly is severe hypotension.[53] Of major importance to the elderly is the fact that hypotensive-induced fainting and dizziness may lead to falling, with the possibility of limb fracture.[53] Elastic stockings may be employed when a severe danger of hypotension is anticipated.[132] The reduced blood pressure may also cause a worsening of the agitated state due to reduced cerebral oxygenation[132] and may also precipitate a heart attack.[53] The incidence of phenothiazine-induced hypotension can be reduced if therapy is initiated at a low dose and then cautiously increased to an acceptable therapeutic level for a given patient.[53] Determination of the proper dosage of phenothiazine therapy can be made more difficult if the individual is also consuming other drugs. The study of Forrest and his associates[39] indicated that alcohol ingestion decreased the metabolism and urinary excretion of chlorpromazine and its metabolites over a twenty-four-hour interval.

Chlorpromazine-induced jaundice is not uncommon in the elderly; in addition, chlorpromazine therapy of the elderly[26] has produced scaling of the skin upon exposure to sunlight. Long-term phenothiazine therapy in the aged has also resulted in corneal defects and increased cataract formation[49, 68] and a few cases of sudden death.[60, 100, 108] Many of the sudden-death victims were found to have lesions of small blood vessels within the heart.[108, 109] Although the various phenothiazines have been successful in the treatment of the young and elderly patients, these problems have limited the usefulness of the phenothiazines in the geriatric population.[133]

Antianxiety Drugs

Benzodiazepines

Chlordiazepoxide (Librium), diazepam (Valium), oxazepam (Serax®): These heavily prescribed drugs belong to a class of compounds known as the *benzodiazepines* and are useful in alleviating symptoms of anxiety, in calming agitation, and in treating withdrawal states from alcohol.[21, 36] Diazepam (Valium) also has properties of a skeletal muscle relaxant.[118] The benzodiazepines have a narrow therapeutic range between a dosage that provides therapeutic effects and one that produces such undesirable side effects as drowsiness, depression, impaired memory, poor coordination, skeletal muscle weakness, and disinhibition.[66, 132] CNS depression and drowsiness are more common with advanced age.[76] The frequency of drowsiness is reported to be almost twice as high in patients over seventy years of age who received Librium as in those under forty years of age.[67] This difference is probably due to decreased metabolism of the drug by the aged liver.

Of some interest is the observation that drowsiness due to benzodiazepines was less prominent among smokers than non-smokers.[67] It is thought that nicotine induces liver enzyme activity, which increases the metabolism of the benzodiazepines in smokers;[67] however, other investigators indicate that smoking did not influence the rate of elimination of diazepam in humans.[76] Thus, the actual mechanism of this effect appears debatable at this time. Benzodiazepine-induced depression is not trivial, since in over 80 percent of 154 patients afflicted with drowsiness, the physician elected to discontinue therapy.[67] It is imperative to recognize the possibility that excessively large daily doses of these compounds may be a deterrent to the geriatric patient who desires to maintain an independent residence in the community.

Antidepressant Drugs

Tricyclic Antidepressants

Imipramine (Tofranil), amitriptyline (Elavil), nortriptyline (Aventyl®), desipramine (Pertofrane®, Norpramin®), doxepin (Sinequan®), and protriptyline (Vivactil®): These drugs belong to an interesting group of compounds, the *tricyclic antidepressants*, and are widely used for the treatment of depression. It has been estimated that approximately 0.4 percent of the adult population will, at some time, be afflicted with a depressive illness that requires some medical attention.[124] In some patients, use of tricyclic antidepressants increases the rate of spontaneous improvement, decreases symptom severity (and the danger of suicide), and promotes social adjustment of the depressed patient.

Tricyclic antidepressant therapy of the elderly necessitates that concern be given for the lower threshold of toxic side effects, some of which may include mental confusion, glaucoma, delayed urination, constipation, decreased gastrointestinal movement, dry mouth, Parkinson-like symptoms, and cardiovascular abnormalities.[101, 132] In an effort to avoid these adverse effects, it has been recommended that the entire daily dose of a tricyclic antidepressant be given at bedtime.[50, 74] However, Prange has indicated that the elderly should not receive an entire daily dose at bedtime, since the increased blood level of the drug may be poorly tolerated in the elderly.[101]

Antimanic Drugs

Lithium carbonate (Lithane®, Lithonate®, and Eskalith®): The manic-depressive patient undergoes episodes of mania (characterized by mood elevation, exaggerated feelings of well-being, and psychomotor activity), which are followed by depression. Lithium carbonate is useful in the treatment of the manic phase of manic-depressive reactions and is also effective against the depressive and manic relapses so common to this illness.[28] Lithium should be used rather cautiously in patients over sixty years of age, however, since the ability of an individual to excrete lithium decreases with age so that the half-life of lithium is significantly prolonged in the elderly.[16, 32] During initiation of lithium therapy, it is recommended to increase the dosage at a less rapid rate in elderly patients and to observe them frequently for evidence of lithium-induced adverse effects.[32] In nongeriatric subjects, serum levels of lithium should be monitored twice a week at the initiation of therapy and at least once per month throughout maintenance therapy.[16] The elderly patient may require more frequent analyses of serum lithium, since mental confusion develops at lower blood levels.[28] The symptoms of lithium toxicity, although rarely fatal, are rather drastic. The subject initially feels faint, lethargic, and experiences sweating, along with a pale and waxy skin. These symptoms are followed by a comatose state, which may be of several days' duration, during which time tremor and contraction of skeletal muscle occur.[1, 129] Spontaneous recovery follows cessation of lithium and initiation of supportive therapy. It is imperative that the patient and family members are aware of the symptoms of lithium toxicity in order to insure prompt professional treatment.

Remarks

Peripheral abnormalities, such as urinary tract infection, cardiovascular and respiratory illnesses, and malnutrition, can produce CNS symptoms of mental confusion, depression, mood changes, memory loss, irritability, and restlessness.[26] In many cases, the use of psychoactive drugs may modify the mental symptoms but have no ameliorative effect on the underlying disease process. In other instances, the ingestion of CNS-acting drugs by the elderly may actually exacerbate, or be the primary cause of, many of the CNS symptoms mentioned above. Accordingly, Learoyd has found that deterioration of the condition of nursing home patients was frequently associated with an increase in the dosage and variety of drugs given. In 20 percent of the patients transferred from a nursing home to a psychogeriatric unit, rapid improvement occurred upon cessation of medication.[81]

CARDIOVASCULAR DRUGS

Antihypertensive Drugs

Hypertension, or high blood pressure, is a rather familiar companion of the aged in view of the report that, in the sixty-five-to-seventy-four-year age-group, 16.3 percent of white males and 50.2 percent of black males are afflicted with this condition. Moreover, the incidence of hypertension in white and black women was 37.5 and 66.4 percent, respectively.[120] The deleterious effects of arteriosclerosis on the aged heart, brain, and kidneys are exacerbated by hypertension.[131] Several physiological alterations concomitant with advanced age are thought to be involved in the direct correlation between age and incidence of hypertension. There is a significant reduction of renal blood flow, renal function, and cardiac output in elderly men and women.[14]

These alterations are also accompanied by arterial wall calcification[7] and an increased vascular resistance.[23] Reduction of hypertension in both young and elderly subjects appears to be correlated with a reduced incidence of vascular complications and mortality;[8, 96] however, drug-induced side effects are problematic with all antihypertensive therapy but especially in the geriatric patient who is less readily persuaded to accept the side effects associated with such therapy.[7] In many cases, a blood pressure of 200/90 in the elderly is left untreated if there are no symptoms. Therapy is usually initiated in a geriatric patient if the blood pressure exceeds 200/105.[23]

Diuretics

Chlorothiazide (Diuril®), hydrochlorothiazide (HydroDIURIL®), chlorthalidone (Hygroton®), and bendroflumethiazide (Naturetin®): These represent a partial list of the diuretics, which are useful in decreasing an elevated blood pressure. The action of diuretics to increase water loss from the body and to thus decrease blood volume is thought to be secondary to their ability to relax smooth muscle with subsequent reduction of peripheral resistance[22] and blood pressure. Since older subjects have a decreased ability to concentrate urine, diuretic therapy should be initiated at half the usual adult dosage in order to avoid excessive sodium and potassium depletion.[23]

Oral diuretics alone provide adequate reduction of blood pressure in about 40 percent of geriatric patients with mild to moderate hypertension;[120] diastolic pressures greater than 120 are not routinely controlled by oral diuretics, but these agents are valuable in augmenting the effects of other hypertensive drugs such as methyldopa, hydralazine, and guanethidine.[131] Side effects common to most of the diuretics listed above include hypotension, weakness, inflammation of the pancreas and skin, gastrointestinal irritation, reduced potassium content of blood, and various blood disorders.[120] Elderly patients may experience severe postural hypotension and subsequent risk of injury due to falls, since they are more sensitive to diuretic-induced reduction of plasma.

The fact that diuretics cause a greater potassium loss in geriatric patients,[41] coupled with the eccentric dietary habits of the elderly,[22] may require the administration of a potassium supplement. A liquid form of potassium is recommended, since the administration of potassium chloride enteric-coated tablets in combination with a diuretic has resulted in complaints of abdominal discomforts, nausea, diarrhea, and loss of appetite, which is followed by chronic obstruction or perforation of the small intestine.[126]

Reserpine (Serpasil®): Reserpine, which is useful in mild hypertension,[120] is usually less effective in elderly patients.[95] Some of the adverse effects of reserpine include sedation, depression, decreased libido, increased appetite, gastric distress, Parkinson-like rigidity, premature ventricular contraction, and nasal congestion. These side effects represent serious deterrents to the use of reserpine in geriatric patients.[120] Reserpine-induced depression, which has been estimated to occur in up to 18 percent of patients,[89] may become a problem of such magnitude that psychiatric hospitalization of the elderly patient is required.[52,71] This drug-induced depression may be rather insidious, or it may be so subtle that it is apparent only in retrospect upon cessation of therapy.[120] Both the patient and family members should be cognizant of the fact that reserpine-induced depression does not subside for several weeks after cessation of therapy.

Clonidine (Catapres®): Clonidine hydrochloride is an oral antihypertensive agent recently released by the Food and Drug Administration for clinical use in the United States. Clonidine is more effective when combined with an oral diuretic, and this combination has proven successful in treating moderately severe or severe hypertension.[77] The most common side effects of clonidine are rather persistent sedation, dryness of the mouth, and dizziness.[98] Not to be overlooked are depression,[61,84] postural hypotension,[33] impotence,[98] and metallic taste.

A drug-induced impotence in elderly males is often neglected due to feelings of embarrassment or its incorrect interpretation as an inevitable companion of old age.[120] Drowsiness, on the other hand, is so annoying that patients may refuse to continue taking the drug.[90] The abrupt discontinuation of clonidine therapy has resulted in a withdrawal syndrome and a potentially fatal rebound hypertensive crisis.[54,63,133] Planned withdrawal, under the direction of the prescribing physician, should be accomplished over a period of at least one week.[77]

Another academically interesting but therapeutically dangerous possibility should be discussed. Individuals maintained on clonidine therapy who experience mental depression (due to endogenous or drug-induced factors) should not receive a tricyclic antidepressant drug such as imipramine. The simultaneous administration of imipramine-like compounds impairs the hypotensive action of clonidine by blockade of (1) the accumulation of clonidine into nerves or (2) the effect of clonidine on certain nerves of the brain. This drug interaction results in an unacceptable elevated arterial pressure, with the effects being more prominent in the supine rather than the erect position.[13]

Guanethidine (Ismelin®): The chemical norepinephrine is normally released from sympathetic nerves which connect to blood vessels and the heart. Enhanced release of norepinephrine elevates blood pressure by constricting most blood vessels and increasing the rate and force of the heart beat. Guanethidine is valuable in the treatment of severe hypertension by virtue of its ability to decrease the release of norepinephrine from sympathetic nerves. It is thought that this drug should be avoided in elderly hypertensive patients.[7] Hypotensive episodes upon standing, the most dangerous side effect of guanethidine therapy,[131] are relatively rare in the young but may be hazardous in geriatric patients who have atherosclerotic or cerebrovascular disease.[7] Elderly patients should arise slowly and avoid prolonged, immobile standing[120] in an effort to avoid dizziness which, due to a misleading high recumbent blood pressure, may be regarded as an indication of additional hypotensive medication.[7]

Two rather disquieting effects reported with guanethidine therapy are diarrhea (which may occur without warning) and failure of ejaculation.[120] Diarrhea may be controlled by the administration of an anticholinergic drug[131] or over-the-counter antidiarrhea preparations; however, there is no apparent treatment of drug-induced failure of ejaculation. Additional side effects include weakness, nasal congestion, and decreased heart rate. The hypotensive effect of guanethidine is blocked by concurrent therapy with a tricyclic antidepressant drug.

Cardiac Glycosides

Digitalis: *Digitalis* represents several steroid glycosides most commonly obtained from the biennial plants *Digitalis purpurea* and *Digitalis lanata*. Although the overall effects of the digitalis preparations on the heart are quite complex and controversial, it is sufficient to state that the digitalis preparations share a common action to increase the force of myocardial contraction. The various digitalis preparations vary in such parameters as potency, rate of absorption, onset of action, and rates of metabolism and excretion. Digitalis therapy is indicated in the treatment of congestive heart failure and is taken by about 5 percent of the geriatric population.[18]

Digitalis is a difficult drug to administer, since the therapeutic zone between effectiveness and digitoxicity is very narrow; in addition, the elderly are more sensitive to digitalis intoxication, which may actually aggravate congestive heart failure.[56] Such an effect may be due to a decreased excretion rate of digitalis in the elderly, in view of the report that administration of equal doses of digoxin in young and old subjects resulted in twice the blood levels and a longer half-life in older subjects.[18, 34, 111] Another study reported that administration of equal doses of digoxin, which is not metabolized in the liver,[31] to an elderly population resulted in therapeutic serum concentrations of digoxin in geriatric patients with normal renal function but toxic levels in geriatric patients with renal impairment.[127] Hurwitz and Wade have indicated that 28.8 percent of digitalis recipients in the seventy-to-seventy-nine-year age-group experienced signs of toxicity.[64] The above information lends credence to the belief that elderly patients receiving digitalis therapy require substantial supervision; in this regard, Thomas has recommended that elderly patients should be examined at least once a week and has also indicated the need for frequent electrocardiographs.[128] This precaution is further strengthened by several reports indicating that a high correlation exists between hypokalemia (due to diuretics, laxatives, and/or poor diet), ischemic heart disease (which is prevalent in the elderly), and susceptibility to the toxic effects of digitalis.[27, 34, 35]

In nongeriatric subjects, digitalis toxicity normally results in such symptoms as loss of appetite, nausea, vomiting, diarrhea, extra heart beats, and cardiac arrhythmias, any of which serve as an indication to reduce the dose of digitalis. The symptoms of digitoxicity in geriatric patients may differ markedly from those just presented. Instead of the usual nausea and vomiting, the elderly may experience loss of appetite, a brown or yellowish hazy vision, and cardiac arrhythmias which may appear in the absence of other signs of toxicity and may represent the first evidence of digitalis overdose.[41] Of special significance is the report that one-fourth of geriatric digitoxicity victims exhibit no symptoms at all and that proper diagnosis was overlooked for several weeks in 50 percent of digitalis intoxication cases.[56] A decreased heart rate sufficient to produce dizziness and partial or complete heart block has also been observed with digitalization of geriatric individuals.[88] The incidence of ocular side effects due to digitalis has approached 25 percent,[42] the onset varies from days to years,[69] and upon cessation of digitalis therapy, the visual symptoms may clear in several days or may be permanent.[110] Thus, in view of the above information, it was not surprising to learn that, over a three-year period, digoxin was the second leading individual drug involved in drug-induced illness requiring hospitalization.

The report of Marsh and Perlman contains some very important information concerning the self-administration of digoxin by chronically ill patients who live at home.[86] In essence, they found that patients who did not have at least a basic understanding of congestive heart failure took their prescribed digitalis less regularly and were hospitalized more often than patients who did understand the disease. Forty-three percent of sixty patients interviewed failed to take the digitalis as prescribed; in fact, two patients failed to have their digitalis prescriptions filled.

NONPRESCRIPTION ANALGESIC DRUGS

Salicylates

Since the salicylates are contained in hundreds of different proprietary products (plus a substantial number of analgesic prescription drugs), it is impossible to offer a representative list at this time. The more common salicylates include aspirin or acetylsalicylic acid and sodium salicylate.

In view of the estimated 12,000 tons of aspirin consumed annually in the United States,[30] the incidence of aspirin-related adverse effects per patient is rather low.[126] However, due to its frequent use by such a large portion of the population, aspirin has been reported to be the single drug most frequently involved in drug-induced illnesses requiring hospitalization.[19] In 1970, aspirin accounted for approximately 22 percent of all internally administered drug poisoning cases and typically results in about 200 deaths per year in the United States.[30, 83] Many older people, however, are convinced that it is a harmless drug and voluntarily consume large amounts to treat their aches and pains.[41]

Possible side effects due to excessive amounts of aspirin and related compounds are very diverse and include allergic reactions, such as skin eruptions; asthma;[114] increased bleeding time; gastrointestinal symptoms, such as nausea, vomiting, abdominal pain, and gastrointestinal hemorrhage;[102] CNS effects, such as tremor, confusion, drowsiness, dizziness, temporary deafness, and hallucinations;[48, 97] and renal and liver damage.[80, 136, 140] The incidence of allergic reactions to aspirin therapy occur in about 0.2 percent.[83] It is thought that the increased bleeding time is clinically significant only if the patient is also receiving anticoagulant therapy, in which case the dosage of anticoagulant medication should be reduced.[105] The gastrointestinal hemorrhage of aspirin therapy, which ranges from 2 to 6 milliliters (ml) per day in about 70 percent of patients,[121] is not considered clinically significant in most cases.[5, 24] However, large daily doses of aspirin may lead to iron-deficiency anemia in patients with inadequate diets, and occasional blood losses of 100 ml per day have been reported.[121] Scott and his associates have suggested an aspirin-induced loss of 4 ml of blood per day for a year causes a depletion of iron stores;[121] however, Baragar and Duthie provided evidence that the hemoglobin value of arthritic patients who ingested up to 3.9 g of aspirin daily tended to increase slightly over a six-year period.[5] Another study reported aspirin to be the primary factor for iron-deficiency anemia in only a small number of rheumatoid arthritic patients but was the major cause of the anemia in twenty of twenty-six nonarthritic patients who ingested aspirin frequently.[137] Since many older persons routinely take one or several aspirin tablets on an empty stomach before retiring, some physicians have recommended that food should be eaten before taking aspirin and that the tablets should be crushed prior to being swallowed to reduce gastric irritation;[41] however, other investigators are of the opinion that ingestion of aspirin tablets on a full stomach does not reduce bleeding.[121]

It is imperative to mention that ingestion of ethyl alcohol increases the gastrointestinal bleeding produced by salicylates;[44] thus, this problem is not to be overlooked in the geriatric population, which consumes a larger volume of alcoholic beverages than is generally believed. Aspirin and its derivatives should not be withheld from the elderly, but their long-term use should be accompanied by periodic hemoglobin determinations and supplemental iron therapy when appropriate.[121]

Although aspirin has been employed as a therapeutic agent for over one hundred years, the emergence of evidence which described liver damage due to high doses of aspirin did not appear until 1956.[85] The incidence of aspirin-induced liver damage may be greater than previously reported, since there are similarities between the symptoms of salicylate intoxication and hepatitis.[136] It has been reported that approximately 50 percent of patients who ingested 3 to 5 g/day of aspirin, which resulted in blood levels of 20 to 45 mg/100 ml of blood, experienced liver damage not due to drug hypersensitivity.[112, 140] These patients had degenerative changes evident upon liver biopsy. In some cases, the diagnosis of chronic active hepatitis was actually considered.[122] Fortunately, these changes were reversible upon cessation of aspirin therapy but readily reappeared upon subsequent challenge with aspirin.[136] It appears that prolonged administration of aspirin or other salicylates is required to produce hepatotoxicity; in addition, there have been no deaths from salicylate-induced liver damage so far.[140] However, other clinicians have addressed the possibility that continuation of aspirin therapy after initiation of liver damage could result in more severe liver disease and even fatal massive necrosis.[136] Wolfe, Metzger, and Goldstein recommend that salicylate blood levels and liver function be periodically determined in patients who receive chronic high-dose salicylate therapy.[136]

One of the infrequent but more serious side effects of aspirin therapy is the fact that normal therapeutic doses of aspirin may precipitate cardiovascular shock characterized by hypotension when given to patients afflicted with gram-negative rod infections.[20] The aspirin-induced cardiovascular shock syndrome, which occurs more often in the elderly,[20] has been accompanied by abnormal heart beats, mimicking an impending myocardial infarction; however, serial electrocardiograms do not reveal myocardial infarction.[99]

It is interesting to speculate on the mechanism of such a drastic response to a normal therapeutic dose of aspirin. A large portion of circulating salicylates are bound to plasma proteins, notably albumin, so that their pharmacological activity is proportional to the amount of drug that is not bound to plasma protein.[29, 107] Aspirin is bound to protein to a small degree; however, up to 75 percent of plasma aspirin is rapidly deacetylated to form salicylic acid, which is highly bound to plasma protein.[138] There is evidence that a decreased binding of salicylates to serum protein occurs in individuals who are hypersensitive to aspirin[125] and also that some infections may dramatically reduce plasma albumin concentration.[17] Thus, Reynolds and Cluff have suggested that an exaggerated salicylate response may occur in patients with depressed serum albumin, since more of the drug is available to exert its pharmacological activity,[107] which in toxic amounts may consist of circulatory depression.[2, 46]

CONCLUDING REMARKS

In order to keep the plethora of information presented in proper perspective, it is necessary to emphasize that the geriatric population can be successfully treated with most drugs; however, such therapy often requires alteration and individualization of drug dosage in order to obtain the desired therapeutic response and to reduce the incidence of deleterious side effects. Although they are predisposed to a greater incidence of drug-induced side effects, the elderly can be assisted in dealing with this problem through increased involvement of medical personnel (prescribing physician, pharmacist, and nurse) and family members. Even if the proper dose of a prescription drug has been established, the report of Marsh and Perlman, which indicates that patient compliance with prescription directions is proportional to the patient's understanding of the disease process being treated,[86] cannot be overlooked. Thus, it seems logical that if the patient were presented with appropriate basic information concerning the disease process and the drug or drugs prescribed for its treatment (with particular reference to possible side effects), then the opportunity for successful treatment would be enhanced, since recognition and reporting of drug-induced side effects permit adjustment of dosage or drug substitution by the physician and continuation of therapy for the patient. Family members too can play a valuable role in the proper taking of medication by the elderly and also in the recognition and reporting of any drug-induced side effects that may occur.

REFERENCES

1. Agulnik, P. L., Dimascio, A., and Moore, P.: Acute brain syndrome associated with lithium therapy. *Am J Psychiatry, 129*:621-623, 1972.
2. Alexander, W. D. and Smith, G.: Disadvantageous circulatory effects of salicylate in rheumatic fever. *Lancet, 1*:768-771, 1962.
3. Apogi, E.: *Cowdry's Problems of Aging.* Baltimore, Williams & Wilkins, 1952.
4. Ayd, F. J.: Persistent dyskinesia: A neurologic complication of major tranquilizers. *Int Drug Ther Newsletter, 1*:1-4, 1966.
5. Baragar, F. D. and Duthie, J. R.: Importance of aspirin as a cause of anaemia and peptic ulcer in rheumatoid arthritis. *Br Med J, 1*:1106-1109, 1960.
6. Baron, J. H.: Studies of basal peak acid output with an augmented histamine test. *Gut, 4*:136-141, 1963.
7. Bauer, G. E.: Treatment of hypertension in the elderly. *Drugs, 7*:310-318, 1974.
8. Bechgaard, P., Kopp, H., and Neelsen, J.: One thousand hypertensive patients followed from 16 to 22 years. *Acta Med Scand [Suppl], 312*:175, 1956.
9. Bender, A. D.: Pharmacologic aspects of aging: A survey of the effects of increasing age on drug activity in adults. *J Am Geriatr Soc, 12*:114-129, 1964.
10. ———: Effects of age on intestinal absorption: Implications for drug absorption in the elderly. *J Am Geriatr Soc, 16*:1331-1339, 1968.

11. Bondareef, W.: Morphology of the aging nervous system. In Birren, J. E. (Ed.): *Handbook on Aging and the Individual.* Chicago, U of Chicago Pr, 1959.
12. Bland, J.: Regulation of fluid and electrolyte balance in the renal function in adult man. *J Am Geriatr Soc, 1*:233-243, 1953.
13. Briant, R. H., Reid, J. L., and Dollery, C. T.: Interaction between clonidine and desipramine in man. *Br Med J, 1*:522-523, 1973.
14. Brod, J.: Changes of renal function with age. *Schriftenr Med (Brno), 41*:223-229, 1969.
15. Brody, H.: Organization of the cerebral cortex. III. A study of aging in the human cerebral cortex. *J Comp Neurol, 102*:511-556, 1955.
16. Brown, W. T.: The use of lithium carbonate in the treatment of mood disorders. *Can Med Assoc J, 108*:742-752, 1973.
17. Bruce, R. and Alling, E.: Electrophoretic changes in plasma proteins in patients with pneumococcic infections. *Proc Soc Exp Biol Med, 69*:398-404, 1948.
18. Caird, F. I.: Metabolism of digoxin in relation to therapy in the elderly. *Gerontol Clin, 16*:68-74, 1972.
19. Caranasos, G. J., Stewart, R. B., and Cluff, L. E.: Drug-induced illness leading to hospitalization. *JAMA, 228*:713-717, 1974.
20. Carter, M.: Personal communication, 1975.
21. Chesrow, E. J., Kaplitz, S. E., Breme, J. T., Musci, J., and Sabatini, R.: Use of benzodiazepine derivative (Valium). *J Am Geriatr Soc, 10*:667-670, 1962.
22. Conway, J. and Palmers, H.: The vascular effects of thiazide diuretics. *Arch Intern Med, 111*:203-207, 1963.
23. Conway, J. and Sannerstedt, R.: Use and abuse of hypotensive drugs in the elderly. *Postgrad Med, 43*:116-121, 1968.
24. Cooke, A. R.: The role of acid in the pathogenesis of aspirin-induced gastrointestinal erosions and hemorrhage. *Digest Dis, 18*:225-237, 1973.
25. Crane, G. E.: Tardive dyskinesia in patients treated with major neuroleptics: A review of the literature. *Am J Psychiatry, 124*:40-48, 1968.
26. Daniel, R.: Psychotropic drug use and abuse in the aged. *Geriatrics, 25*:144-158, 1970.
27. Davidson, S. and Surawicz, B.: Ectopic beats and atrioventricular conduction disturbances in patients with hypopotassemia. *Arch Intern Med, 120*:280-285, 1967.
28. Davis, J. M., Fann, W. E., El-Yousef, M. K., and Janowsky, D. S.: Clinical problems in treating the aged with psychotropic drugs. In Eisdorfer, C. and Fann, W. E. (Eds.): *Psychopharmacology and Aging.* New York, Plenum Pr, 1973.
29. Davison, C. and Smith, P. K.: The binding of salicylic acid and

related substances to purified proteins. *J Pharmacol Exp Ther,* 133:161-170, 1961.
30. Davison, C. and Mandel, G.: Non-narcotic analgesics and antipyretics. I. Salicylates. In DiPalma, J. R. (Ed.): *Drill's Pharmacology In Medicine,* 4th ed. New York, McGraw-Hill, 1971.
31. DeGraff, A. C.: Drug therapy of cardiovascular disease. *Geriatrics,* 29:51-54, 1974.
32. deGroot, M. H. L.: The clinical uses of psychotherapeutic drugs in the elderly. *Drugs,* 8:132-138, 1974.
33. Ebringer, A., Doyle, A. E., Dawborn, J. K., Johnston, C. I., and Mashford, M. L.: The use of clonidine (Catapres) in the treatment of hypertension. *Med J Aust,* 57, 1:524-527, 1970.
34. Ewy, G. A., Kapadia, G. G., Yao, L., Lullin, M., and Marcus, F. I.: Digoxin metabolism in the elderly. *Circulation,* 39:449-453, 1969.
35. Ewy, G. A. and Marcus, F. I.: Digitalis therapy in the aged. *Gen Practitioner,* 1:81-85, 1970.
36. Exton-Smith, A. N., Hodkinson, H. M., Cromie, B. W., and Curwen, M. P.: Controlled comparison of four sedative drugs in elderly patients. *Br Med J,* 2:1037-1040, 1963.
37. Fahn, S., Libsch, L. R., and Cutler, R. W.: Monoamines in the human neostriatum: Topographic distribution in normals and in Parkinson's disease and their role in akinesia, rigidity, chorea, and tremor. *J Neurol Sci,* 14:427-455, 1971.
38. Forner, D. and Verzar, F.: The age parameter of pharmacologic activity. *Experientia,* 17:421-422, 1961.
39. Forrest, F. M., Forrest, I. S., and Finkle, B. S.: Alcohol-chlorpromazine interaction in psychiatric patients. *Agressologie,* 13:67-74, 1972.
40. Friedman, S. A., Raizner, A. E., Rosen, H., Solomon, N. A., and Sy, W.: Functional defects in the aging kidney. *Ann Intern Med,* 76:41-45, 1972.
41. Friend, D. G.: Drug therapy and the geriatric patient. *Clin Pharmacol Ther,* 2:832-836, 1961.
42. Gerber, M.: Disturbances of vision caused by digitalis preparations. *J Am Geriatr Soc,* 5:668-670, 1957.
43. Gibson, I.: Barbiturate delirium. *Practitioner,* 197:345-347, 1966.
44. Goulston, K. and Cooke, A. R.: Alcohol, aspirin and gastrointestinal bleeding. *Br Med J,* 4:664-665, 1968.
45. Granerus, A., Goran, S., and Svanborg, A.: Clinical analysis of factors influencing L-dopa treatment of Parkinson's syndrome. *Acta Med Scand,* 192:1-11, 1972.
46. Granville-Grossman, K. L., and Sergeant, H. G. S.: Pulmonary edema due to salicylate intoxication. *Lancet,* 1:575-577, 1960.
47. Greenblatt, D. J., Shader, R. I., and DiMascio, A.: Extrapyramidal defects. In Shader, R. I. and DiMascio, A. (Eds.): *Psychotropic Drug Side Effects: Clinical and Theoretical Perspectives.* Baltimore, Williams & Wilkins, 1970.

48. Greer, H. D., Ward, H. P., and Corbin, K. B.: Chronic salicylate intoxication in adults. *JAMA, 193*:555-558, 1965.
49. Greiner, A. C. and Berry, K.: Skin pigmentation and corneal and lens opacities with prolonged chlorpromazine therapy. *Can Med Assoc J, 90*:663-665, 1964.
50. Haider, I.: A single daily dose of a new form of amitriptyline in depressive illness. *Br J Psychiatry, 120*:521-522, 1972.
51. Hall, M. R. P.: Adverse drug reactions in the elderly. *Gerontol Clin, 16*:144-150, 1974.
52. Halpern, M. M.: Clinical management of hypertension in the older patient. *J Am Geriatr Soc, 9*:48-57, 1961.
53. Hamilton, L. D.: Aged brain and the phenothiazines. *Geriatrics, 21*:131-138, 1966.
54. Hansson, L., Hunyor, S. N., Julius, S., and Hoobler, S. W.: Blood pressure crisis following withdrawal of clonidine (Catapres, Catapresan), with special reference to arterial and urinary catecholamine levels and suggestions for acute management. *Am Heart J, 85*:605-610, 1973.
55. Heider, C. H. and Brest, A. N.: Renal insufficiency in the aged. *Geriatrics, 18*:489-493, 1963.
56. Herrmann, G. R.: Digitoxicity in the aged. *Geriatrics, 21*:109-122, 1966.
57. Himwich, H. E.: Research in medical aspects of aging. *Geriatrics, 17*:89-97, 1962.
58. Hogben, C. A. M., Schanker, L. S., Tocco, D. J., and Brodie, B. B.: Absorption of drugs from the stomach. II. The human. *J Pharmacol Exp Ther, 120*:540-545, 1957.
59. Hogben, C. A. M., Tocco, D. J., Brodie, B. B., and Schanker, L. S.: On the mechanism of intestinal absorption of drugs. *J Pharmacol Exp Ther, 125*:275-282, 1959.
60. Hollister, L. E. and Kosek, J. C.: Sudden death during treatment with phenothiazine derivatives. *JAMA, 192*:1035-1038, 1965.
61. Holman, R. B., Shillito, E., and Vogt, M.: Sleep induced by clonidine. (2-(2,6-dichlorophenylamino)-2-imidazoline hydrochloride). *Br J Pharmacol, 43*:685-695, 1971.
62. Hornykiewicz, O.: Dopamine and brain function. *Pharmacol Rev, 18*:925-964, 1966.
63. Hunyor, S. N., Hansson, L., Harrison, T. S., and Hoobler, S. W.: Effects of clonidine withdrawal: Possible mechanisms and suggestions for management. *Br Med J, 2*:209-211, 1973.
64. Hurwitz, N. and Wade, O. L.: Intensive hospital monitoring of adverse reactions to drugs. *Br Med J, 1*:531-536, 1969.
65. Jacobson, E.: Psychopharmacology and aging in age with a future.

Proceedings of the Sixth International Congress of Gerontology. Amsterdam, Excerpta Medica Foundation, 1963.
66. Janke, W. and Debus, G.: Experimental studies on antianxiety agents with normal subjects: Methodological considerations and review of the main effects. In Efron, D. H. (Ed.): *Psychopharmacology: A Review of Progress, 1957-1967.* Public Health Service Publ. No. 1863, Washington, D.C., U.S. Govt Print Office, 1968.
67. Jick, H.: Clinical depression of the central nervous system due to diazepam and chlordiazepoxide in relation to cigarette smoking and age. *N Engl J Med, 288*:277-280, 1973.
68. Johnson, A. W. and Buffaloe, W. J.: Chlorpromazine epithelial keratopathy. *Arch Ophthalmol, 76*:664-667, 1966.
69. Katz, L. N. and Wise, W.: Oral single-dose digitalization with digitalis leaf and digitaline "Nativelle." *Am Heart J, 30*:125-133, 1945.
70. Keenan, R. E.: The Eaton collaborative study of levodopa therapy in Parkinsonism: A summary. *Neurology, 20*:46-59, 1971.
71. Keyes, J. W.: Problems in drug management in cerebrovascular disorders in geriatric patients. *J Am Geriatr Soc, 13*:118-124, 1965.
72. Klawans, H. L. and Garvin, J. S.: Preliminary observations on the treatment of Parkinsonism with L-dopa: A study of 105 patients. *Dis Nerv Syst, 30*:737-746, 1969.
73. Klawans, H., Ilahi, M. M., and Shenker, D.: Theoretical implications of the use of L-dopa in Parkinsonism. *Acta Neurol Scand, 46*:409-441, 1970.
74. Klein, D. F. and Davis, J. M.: *Diagnosis and Drug Treatment of Psychiatric Disorders.* Baltimore, Williams & Wilkins, 1969.
75. Kline, N. S.: On the rarity of "irreversible" oral dyskinesias following phenothiazines. *Am J Psychiatry, 124*:48-54, 1968.
76. Klotz, U., Avant, G. R., Hoyumpa, A., Schneker, S., and Wilkinson, G. R.: The effects of age and liver disease on the disposition and elimination of diazepam in adult man. *J Clin Invest, 55*:347-359, 1975.
77. Kosman, M. E.: Evaluation of chonidine hydrochloride (Catapres): A new antihypertensive agent. *JAMA, 233*:174-176, 1975.
78. Kurland, L. T.: Epidemiology, incidence, geographic distribution and genetic considerations. In Fields, W. S. (Ed.): *Pathogenesis and Treatment of Parkinsonism.* Springfield, Thomas, 1958.
79. Langrell, H. M. and Joseph, C.: Status of the clinical evaluation of levodopa in the treatment of Parkinson's disease and syndrome. *Clin Pharmacol Ther, 12*:323-331, 1971.
80. Lawson, A. A. H. and MacLean, N.: Renal disease and drug therapy in rheumatoid arthritis. *Ann Rheum Dis, 25*:441-449, 1966.

81. Learoyd, B. M.: Psychotropic drugs in the elderly patient. *Med J Aust*, 1:1131-1132, 1972.
82. Lehmann, H. E.: Psychopharmacological aspects of geriatric medicine. In Gaitz, C. M. (Ed.): *Aging and the Brain*. New York, Plenum Pr, 1972.
83. Levine, R. R.: *Pharmacology, Drug Actions and Reactions*. Boston, Little, Brown & Co., 1973.
84. MacDougall, A. I., Addis, G. J., Mackay, N., Dymock, I. W., Tarpie, A. G. G., Ballingal, D. L. K., MacLennan, W. J., Whiting, B., and MacArthur, J. G.: Treatment of hypertension with clonidine. *Br Med J*, 3:440-442, 1970.
85. Manso, C., Taranta, A., and Mydrick, J.: Effect of aspirin administration on serum glutamic oxaloacetic and glutamic pyruvic transaminases in children. *Proc Soc Exp Biol Med*, 93:84-85, 1956.
86. Marsh, W. W. and Perlman, L. V.: Understanding congestive heart failure and self-administration of digoxin. *Geriatrics*, 27:65-70, 1972.
87. Martin, W. E., Loewenson, R. B., Bilck, M. K., Resch, J. A., and Baker, A. B.: Long-term treatment of Parkinson's disease with levodopa. *J Chronic Dis*, 27:77-93, 1974.
88. Master, A.: Treatment of coronary disease with special reference to older people. *J Am Geriatr Soc*, 9:163-177, 1961.
89. *Med Lett Drugs Ther*, 14:35-36, 1972.
90. *Med Lett Drugs Ther*, 17:45, 1975.
91. Miller, E.: Deanol in the treatment of levodopa-induced dyskinesias. *Neurology*, 24:116-119, 1974.
92. Miller, E. M. and Nieburg, H. A.: L-tryptophan in the treatment of levodopa-induced psychiatric disorders. *Dis Nerv Syst*, 35:20-23, 1974.
93. Mitchell, A. D. and Velk, W. L.: Renal function in the aged. *Geriatrics*, 8:263-266, 1953.
94. Mones, R. J., Elizan, T. S., and Siegel, G. J.: Evaluation of L-dopa therapy in Parkinson's disease. *NY State J Med*, 70:2309, 1970.
95. Moyer, J. H., Kinard, S. A., Conner, P. K., and Dennis, E.: Drug therapy of hypertension in the elderly patient. *Geriatrics*, 11:527-542, 1956.
96. Moyer, J. H., Heider, C., Pevey, K., and Ford, R. V.: The effect of treatment on the vascular deterioration associated with hypertension with particular emphasis on renal function. *Am J Med*, 24:177-192, 1958.
97. Myers, E. N., Bernstein, J. M., and Fostiropolous, G.: Salicylate-induced disease, salicylate ototoxicity. *N Engl J Med*, 273:587-590, 1965.
98. Onesti, G., Bock, K. D., Heimsoth, V., Kim, K. E., and Merguet, P.:

Clonidine: A new antihypertensive agent. *Am J Cardiol,* 28:74-83, 1971.
99. Paul, B. N.: Salicylate poisoning in the elderly: Diagnostic pitfalls. *J Am Geriatr Soc,* 20:387-390, 1972.
100. Peele, R. and von Loetzen, I. S.: Phenothiazine deaths: A critical review. *Am J Psychiatry,* 130:306-308, 1973.
101. Prange, A. J.: The use of antidepressant drugs in the elderly patient. In Eisdorfer, C. and Fann, W. E. (Eds.): *Psychopharmacology and Aging.* New York, Plenum Pr, 1973.
102. Prescott, L. F.: Antipyretic analgesic drugs. In Meyler, L. and Herxheimer, A. (Eds.): *Side Effects of Drugs.* Baltimore, Williams & Wilkins, 1968.
103. Prien, R. F., Levine, J., and Cole, J. O.: Indications for high dose chlorpromazine therapy in chronic schizophrenia. *Dis Nerv Syst,* 31:739-745, 1970.
104. Proudfoot, A. T. and Wright, N.: The physical consequences of self-poisoning by the elderly. *Gerontol Clin,* 14:25-31, 1972.
105. Quick, A. J. and Clesceri, L.: Influence of acetylsalicylic acid and salicylamide on the coagulation of blood. *J Pharmacol Exp Ther,* 128:95-98, 1960.
106. Reveno, W. S., Bauer, R. B., and Rosenbaum, H.: L-dopa for Parkinsonism. *Geriatrics,* 28:86-88, 1973.
107. Reynolds, R. C. and Cluff, L. E.: Interaction of serum and sodium salicylate: Changes during acute infection and its influence on pharmacological activity. *Bull Johns Hopkins Hosp,* 105:278-290, 1960.
108. Richardson, H. L., Graupner, K. I., and Murphree, O. D.: Myocardial arteriolar alterations in patients on phenothiazines. *Circulation [Suppl 2],* 32:179, 1965.
109. Richardson, H. L., Graupner, K. I., and Richardson, M. E.: Intramyocardial lesion in patients dying suddenly and unexpectedly. *JAMA,* 195:254-260, 1966.
110. Robertson, D. M., Hollenhorst, R. W., and Callahan, J. A.: Ocular manifestations of digitalis toxicity. *Arch Ophthalmol,* 76:640-645, 1966.
111. Rosenberg, J. M. and Mann, K.: Factors that modify drug activity and patient response. *Drug Intell Clin Pharm,* 7:346-350, 1973.
112. Russell, A. S., Sturge, R. A., and Smith, M. A.: Serum transaminase during salicylate therapy. *Br Med J,* 2:428-429, 1971.
113. Salter, W. T.: Use of drugs for older people. *Geriatrics,* 7:317-323, 1952.
114. Samter, M. and Beers, R. F.: Intolerance to aspirin: Clinical studies and consideration of its pathogenesis. *Ann Intern Med,* 68:975-983, 1968.

115. Schanker, L. S., Shore, P. A., Brodie, B. B., and Hogben, C. A. M.: Absorption of drugs from the stomach. I. The Rat. *J Pharmacol Exp Ther, 120*:528-539, 1957.
116. Schanker, L. S.: Passage of drugs across body membranes. *Pharmacol Rev, 14*:501-530, 1962.
117. Schmidt, W. R. and Jarcho, L. W.: Persistent dyskinesia following phenothiazine therapy. *Arch Neurol, 14*:360-377, 1966.
118. Schmidt, R. F., Vogel, M. E., and Zimmerman, M.: Die Wirkung von Diazepam auf die parasynaptische Hemmung und andere ruckenmarsk Reflexe. *Naunyn Schmiedebergs Arch Exp Pathol Pharmacol, 258*:69-82, 1976.
119. Schwartz, D.: The elderly patient and his medications. *Geriatrics, 20*:517-520, 1965.
120. Schwid, S. A. and Gifford, R. W.: The use and abuse of antihypertensive drugs in the aged. *Geriatrics, 22*:172-182, 1967.
121. Scott, J. T., Porter, I. H., Lewis, S. M., and Dixon, A. St. J.: Studies of gastrointestinal bleeding caused by corticosteroids, salicylates, and other analgesics. *Q J Med, 118*:167-188, 1961.
122. Seaman, W. E., Ishak, K. G., and Plotz, P. H.: Aspirin induced hepatotoxicity in patients with systemic lupus erythrematosus. *Ann Intern Med, 80*:1-8, 1974.
123. Shepherd, M., Lader, M., and Lader, S.: Central nervous system depressants. In Meyler, L. and Herxheimer, A. (Eds.): *Side Effects of Drugs*. Baltimore, Williams & Wilkins, 1968.
124. Silverman, C.: The epidemiology of depression: A review. *Am J Psychiatry, 124*:883-891, 1968.
125. Storm van Leeuwen, W. and Drizmal, H.: Uber des Bindungs fahigkeit des Blutes fur Salicylsaure in Zusammenhang mit uberemfindlichkeit gegen Salicylsaure. *Naunyn Schmiedebergs Arch Exp Pathol Pharmakol, 102*:218-225, 1924.
126. Sun, D. C. H.: Iatrogenic gastrointestinal diseases in the aged. *Geriatrics, 27*:89-95, 1972.
127. Taylor, B. B., Kennedy, R. D., and Caird, F. I.: Digoxin studies on the elderly. *Age Aging, 3*:79-84, 1974.
128. Thomas, J. H.: The use and abuse of digitalis in the elderly. *Gerontol Clin, 13*:285-295, 1971.
129. Van Der Velde, C. D.: Toxicity of lithium carbonate in elderly patients. *Am J Psychiatry, 127*:1075-1077, 1971.
130. Vernon, S.: Nocturia in the elderly male. *J Am Geriatr Soc, 6*:411-414, 1958.
131. Vidt, D. G.: An approach to the medical treatment of hypertension in the aged. *Geriatrics, 24*:120-129, 1969.
132. Webb, W. L.: The use of psychopharmacological drugs in the aged. *Geriatrics, 26*:95-103, 1971.

133. Webster, J., Jeffers, A., Galloway, D. B., and Petrie, J. C.: Withdrawal of antihypertensive therapy. *Lancet,* 2:1381-1382, 1974.
134. Williams, G. R.: Morbidity and mortality with Parkinsonism. *J Neurosurg [Suppl], 24*:138, 1966.
135. Williams, R. T.: Detoxification mechanisms in man. *Clin Pharmacol Ther, 4*:234-254, 1963.
136. Wolfe, J. D., Metzger, A. L., and Goldstein, R. C.: Aspirin hepatitis. *Ann Intern Med, 80*:74-76, 1974.
137. Wood, P. N. H. and Wilson, C. H.: Iron-deficiency anemia in rheumatoid arthritis, and the role of aspirin-induced gastrointestinal bleeding in the pathogenesis. *Arthritis Rheum,* 7:354, 1964.
138. Woodbury, D. M.: Analgesic-antipyretics, anti-inflammatory agents, and inhibitors of uric acid synthesis. In Goodman, L. S. and Gilman, A. (Eds.): *The Pharmacologic Basis of Therapeutics,* 4th ed. New York, Macmillan, 1970.
139. Yahr, M. D., Duvoisin, R. C., Schear, M. J., Barrett, R. E., and Hoehn, M. M.: Treatment of Parkinsonism with levodopa. *Arch Neurol, 21*:343-354, 1969.
140. Zimmerman, H. J.: Aspirin-induced hepatic injury. *Ann Intern Med, 80*:103-105, 1974.

Chapter 6

DRUG INTERACTIONS IN THE ELDERLY*
DONALD E. CADWALLADER, PH.D.

As PEOPLE GROW OLDER, they demonstrate a need for multiple-drug therapy to treat a variety of disease states. The ingestion of numerous drugs coupled with the possible decrease in physiological capabilities make the elderly particularly susceptible to adverse drug reactions and drug-drug interactions. Age is an important physiologic factor in the consideration of drug reactions and interactions. Studies indicate that there is an increased incidence of adverse drug reactions in geriatric patients, and an estimate by Melmon[2] suggests that the risk of drug reaction in patients sixty to seventy years old is almost double that in adults thirty to forty years old. Although renal and hepatic function in the elderly may be diminished, there is no evidence that these factors in general are responsible for increased drug sensitivity. It is the aging process by its very nature that is responsible for the high incidence and severity of drug reactions and interactions in the elderly. This theme is developed in Figure 6-1. The aging process leads to many different disease states, some acute, some chronic, and one disease state possibly leading to another. Diabetes, arthritis and bursitis, glaucoma, emphysema, ulcers and other gastrointestinal (GI) disorders, urinary tract problems, high blood pressure, atherosclerosis, heart failure, and stroke are only some of the diseases associated with advanced years. It is a lucky older person that suffers only one or two of these conditions. In addition to this, the eyes are getting weak, hearing is failing, and constipation is becoming a way of life. Figure 6-1

---

* The author would like to thank Roche Laboratories, Nutley, New Jersey, for permission to reproduce figures and tables from the author's monograph, *Biopharmaceutics and Drug Interactions*, 2nd ed. Roche Scientific Monographs, 1974.

shows that multiple diseases, in fact, many single diseases (high blood pressure, for example), lead to multiple-drug therapy; the more drugs a patient takes into the body, the greater the chances of adverse drug reactions and interactions occurring. These chances increase geometrically, and the incidences of side effects, allergies, and idiosyncrasies also increase. A major cause of adverse drug reactions is drug-drug interactions. Drug-drug interaction means that one drug modifies the action of another drug.

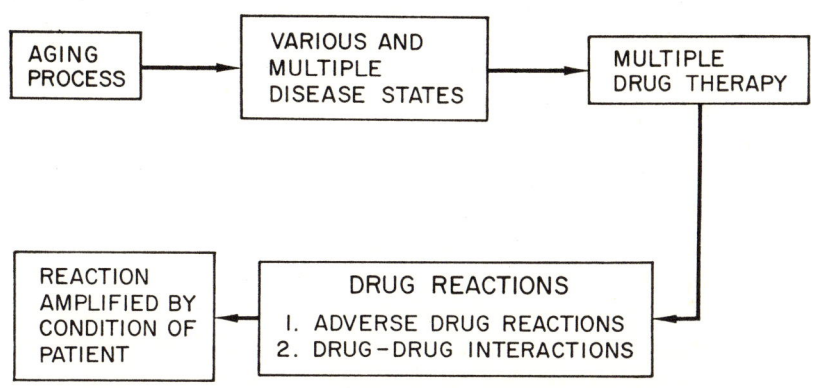

Figure 6-1. Multiple-drug use and adverse reactions in the aged.

The geriatric patient, because of a general debilitated condition, likely has stronger reactions to drug therapy than a younger adult. Instead of a few black-and-blue marks from anticoagulant therapy, the elderly patient might develop internal bleeding. Instead of just a dry mouth from taking antispasmodics, urinary retention might result. Instead of a rise in blood pressure from a drug reaction, hypertensive crises might develop.

Because of the large variety and number of drugs used by the elderly population, drug-drug interactions are an important and growing problem. The purpose of this discussion is to acquaint the reader with the basic problems, principles, and mechanisms of drug-drug interactions. *Drug interactions occur when the effects of one drug are modified by the prior or simultaneous administration of another drug.* In such interactions, the effect of a drug vital to the patient's therapy may be decreased or increased by another drug. In recent years, the explosion of information on drug interactions has made all health professionals well aware of their occurrence and possible danger. There are several reasons for the increased evidence of drug interactions:

1. Drug potency—Many drugs used today are very potent and are used near their toxic levels (the therapeutic index of the drug is low). Also, many drugs have powerful side effects.
2. Multiple-drug use—Older patients not only typically receive several prescription drugs from their physicians for the treatment of multiple conditions but are more than ever exercising their right to treat themselves with nonprescription over-the-counter drugs.
3. Use of medical specialists—In an era of specialization, many older patients see several physicians concurrently, none of whom may be aware of the others' involvement with the patient or drug prescriptions.
4. Better understanding of drug actions—Not every adverse reaction is now blamed on allergies or idiosyncrasies.
5. Better reporting of adverse reactions—Recent reports on research conducted in hospital emergency rooms have documented a significant acute drug reaction problem among older people.

A presentation concerning the problem and principles of unintended drug interactions is best approached by following the drug as it travels into, about, and out of the body. Discussion will concern drug absorption, distribution, metabolism, and excretion. What happens after a drug is taken into the body? When a drug is administered orally, it first must be dissolved in the gastrointestinal fluids before it can pass across the membranes into the systemic circulation. The drug is then distributed to various parts of the body where it may be stored, metabolized, exert a pharmacologic effect, or be excreted. It is *absorption* that determines how much of the drug enters the bloodstream from the site of administration. *Distribution* determines how much of the drug reaches the site of action. *Metabolism,* or *biotransformation,* regulates the conversion of drugs into metabolites that are generally less active than the parent drug. Finally, *excretion* removes the drug or its metabolites from the body, principally by urine. Unintended drug reactions (*drug interactions*) may occur during any one of these processes.

DRUG INTERACTIONS DURING ABSORPTION

The oral route is the most common way of administering drugs because of its convenience and safety. Fortunately, most drugs are readily absorbed from the GI tract, especially from the small intestine with its vast capillary bed and blood supply. Some drugs, however, are destroyed by GI fluids and enzymes or are not absorbed across the membranes. For example, heparin must be given by injection because it is destroyed by GI fluids. Streptomycin must be given by injection for treating systemic infections, since it is not absorbed by the GI tract.

What about drug-drug interactions during absorption? Substances such as charcoal and kaolin are used as antidotes and antidiarrheals because of their adsorptive properties. (Adsorption, as opposed to absorption, refers to the property of binding or fusing one substance with another.) However, when these substances are administered concurrently with certain drugs, there is the possibility of drug interactions that may result in reduced availability of the active ingredients. Figure 6-2 shows how kaolin pectin mixture (Kaopectate®) interferes with the absorption of lincomycin (Lincocin®). For example, when the Kaopectate is taken either two hours before or after the Lincocin, the absorptive capacity of the Lincocin is somewhat impaired. However, when the two drugs are taken simultaneously, the serum concentration of the Lincocin is dramatically reduced. A large portion of the antibiotic is apparently adsorbed on the kaolin and passes through the GI tract without being absorbed into the bloodstream.

Complexation of tetracycline antibiotics may occur when these drugs are administered along with aluminum, magnesium, and calcium antacid products. Figure 6-3 illustrates the greatly decreased bioavailability of demeclocycline hydrochloride (Declomycin®) when it is administered with aluminum hydroxide gel and also with milk. Ferrous sulfate has also been shown to impair the absorption of tetracycline antibiotics. A large number

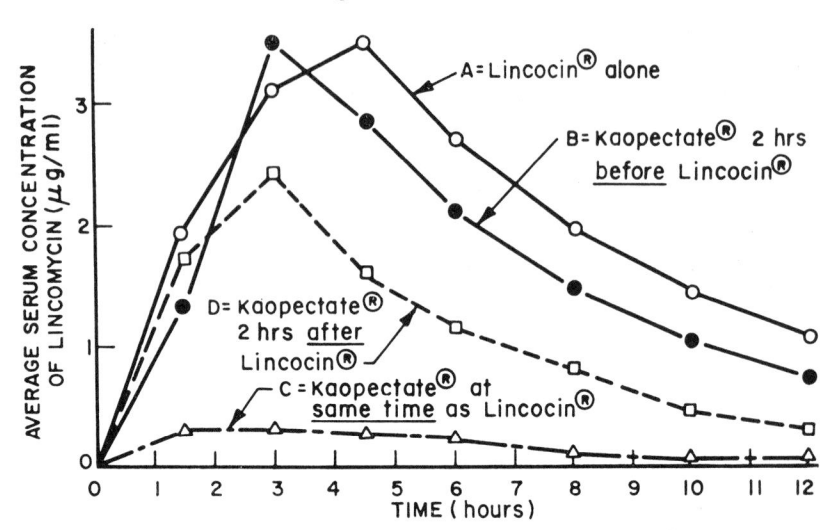

Figure 6-2. Average serum concentrations of lincomycin following a 0.5 g dose of lincomycin in capsule dosage form. From J. G. Wagner, Design and Analysis of Biopharmaceutical Studies in Man. *Canadian Journal of Pharmaceutical Sciences*, 1:55-68, 1966. Courtesy of The Canadian Pharmaceutical Association, Toronto, Ontario.

of geriatric patients are on antacid therapy, sippy diets, and iron therapy and, if the situation arises, should be advised not to take their drugs concurrently with tetracycline antibiotics.

Cholestyramine (Questran®) is a resin that is used to tie up bile salts in the GI tract as a means of reducing cholesterol in the body, and it is used in treating hypercholesterolemia. The drug also complexes (combines) with many drugs and prevents their absorption. It is recommended that resin drugs be given several hours after administration of other drugs.

The gastrointestinal absorption of drugs may be influenced by the presence of food, so the time of administration could be an important consideration when certain drugs are prescribed. Figure 6-4 depicts the average levels in serum after administration of dicloxacillin (Dynapen®) capsules, on a fasting stomach, one hour before a standard meal, and with a standard meal. The penicillin-type antibiotic showed the greatest availability when it was administered on a fasting stomach. It is important that patients take their medications exactly as instructed, e.g. before

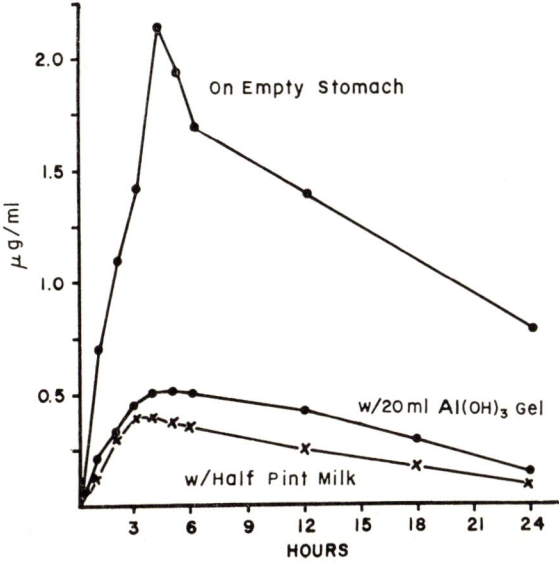

Figure 6-3. Serum concentrations after a single oral dose of 300 mg of demeclocycline hydrochloride. From J. Scheiner and W. A. Altemeier, Experimental Study of Factors Inhibiting Absorption and Effective Therapeutic Levels of Declomycin. *Surgery, Gynecology & Obstetrics, 114*:9-14, 1962. By permission of *Surgery, Gynecology & Obstetrics*.

meals, after meals, and first thing in the morning, etc. There usually is a good reason for giving instructions that maximize the benefits the patient receives from the drug.

DRUG INTERACTIONS DURING TRANSPORT

The distribution of drugs is mainly by the blood plasma, which takes the drug to sites of action, metabolism, and excretion. Most drugs are not very soluble in plasma and are carried in the blood as complexes bound to plasma proteins. Some drugs are more likely to be bound than others, and some compounds are more strongly bound than others. When a drug is bound up in complexes, it is pharmacologically inert. Drug action depends on the adsorption of the free drug by an active receptor site (these are cells or cell surfaces which form molecular bonds with drug molecules), and, therefore, a response to a drug is

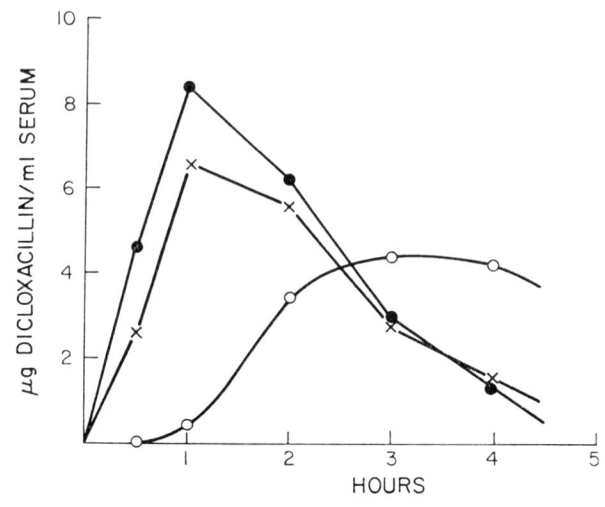

Figure 6-4. Average levels of dicloxacillin activity in serum of adults receiving a 250 mg capsule after an overnight fast (●), one hour before a standard breakfast (x), and with breakfast (o). From J. T. Doluisio, J. C. La Piana, G. R. Wilkinson, and L. W. Dittert, Pharmacokinetic Interpretation of Dicloxacillin Levels in Serum after Extravascular Administration. In G. L. Hobby (Ed.), *Antimicrobial Agents and Chemotherapy—1969-1970*. Courtesy of The American Society for Microbiology, Bethesda, Maryland.

determined in part by the concentration of free drug in the plasma.

If two drugs are given together or one drug is given after another, the one that is more strongly bound is tied up on the protein binding sites, and the less strongly bound drug is free in the bloodstream. The increase in plasma concentration of the free drug causes an increase in this drug's activity, and an overdose can possibly occur. An example of this interaction, which is of clinical importance, is the displacement of coumarin-type anticoagulants by salicylates and Butazolidin®-type drugs which can give high blood levels of anticoagulant and may possibly lead to hemorrhaging.

Some interactions that may occur during transport of drugs in the body are presented in Table 6-I. Sulfonamides, salicylates, and phenylbutazone derivatives are very strongly bound drugs and displace many different moderately bound drugs.

TABLE 6-I
DRUG INTERACTIONS DURING TRANSPORT

Strongly Bound Drug (A)	Moderately Bound Drug (B)	Possible Effect Due to Increased Concentration of B
Sulfonamides (long-acting) Phenylbutazone (Butazolidin) Salicylates	Tolbutamide (Orinase)	Hypoglycemia
Oxyphenylbutazone (Tandearil®) Phenylbutazone Sulfinpyrazone (Anturane®)	Warfarin (Panwarfin®, Coumadin®)	Hemorrhage
Sulfonamides Salicylates	Methotrexate	Cytopenia, blood dyscrasias
Quinacrine (Atabrine®)	Pamaquin	GI distress, anemias
Ethacrynic acid (Edecrin®)	Oral antidiabetics	Hypoglycemia

DRUG INTERACTIONS BY ACCELERATED METABOLISM

The ability of the body to transform drugs into water-soluble metabolites is a very important factor. Without these biotransformations, a drug could be circulated in the body for the lifetime of the patient. There are many enzymatic-metabolic reactions. The details of these chemical reactions will not be discussed, but two important facts about them should be emphasized. First, the transformations usually, but not always, result in inactivation of the drug. Second, the metabolites are more water-soluble than the original drugs, allowing them to be easily eliminated by the kidneys.

Biotransformation of drugs takes place mainly in the liver, and the enzyme systems are located in the hepatic endoplasmic reticulum, the location of the microsomes. It is these microsomal enzymes that catalyze the drug biotransformations. The activity of the enzyme process can be greatly influenced by the administration of certain drugs; the enzyme activity can be increased or decreased.

Prior treatment of experimental animals with various drugs has been shown to increase the rate of metabolism and to shorten the duration of action for subsequent drugs administered. This same type of phenomenon occurs in humans. Chronic administration of one drug can reduce the pharmacologic activity of itself or another drug by stimulating its metabolic breakdown. This effect, produced by increasing the amount of drug metabolizing enzymes in the liver microsomes, is called *enzyme induction*. Some of the classes of drugs which enhance metabolism are the sedative-hypnotics, tranquilizers, analgesics, antihistamines, and oral antidiabetic agents. Phenobarbital, one of the most widely used drugs, is probably the most notorious of the enzyme-inducing drugs.

As a result of increased metabolism, larger-than-usual amounts of the drug would have to be administered to obtain the desired pharmacological response. For example, there are several possible implications of the interaction produced by concurrent administration of phenobarbital and bishydroxycoumarin (Dicumarol®). Because of the enzyme induction effect of phenobarbital, the anticoagulant effect is reduced, and larger-than-usual amounts of bishydroxycoumarin would have to be administered to obtain adequate anticoagulant action. However, if the sedative is stopped and the anticoagulant continued at the adjusted higher dosage, the enzyme-stimulating effect ceases. Then the anticoagulant is not metabolized as fast, and hemorrhaging may result. This problem can be readily detected and corrected in a hospital or clinical environment where the patient's blood clotting time is monitored every day and dosage adjustments made if necessary. However, when the patient is at home and not under constant supervision, a clinically dangerous situation may occur.

DRUG INTERACTIONS BY INHIBITED METABOLISM

A few drug reactions are based on inhibition of metabolism of certain drugs by other drugs. How this occurs is not well understood. The result of such interactions is an increase in the duration and intensity of pharmacologic activity. For example, bishydroxycoumarin may inhibit the metabolism of tolbutamide (Orinase®), and the result could be a high level of hypoglycemic agent, leading to the lowering of blood sugar to dangerous levels. Figure 6-5 illustrates how the concurrent administration of two drugs may result in two different types of drug interactions at the same time. Tolbutamide displaces the anticoagulant from protein binding sites, thereby increasing the anticoagulant activity.

↑ ANTICOAGULANT EFFECT

BISHYDROXYCOUMARIN

DISPLACES ANTICOAGULANT   INHIBITS METABOLISM

TOLBUTAMIDE

↑ HYPOGLYCEMIC EFFECT

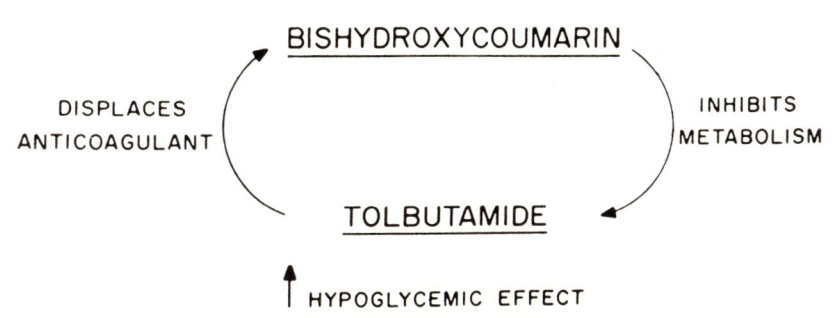

Figure 6-5. Interactions between bishydroxycoumarin and tolbutamide which might occur in man. From H. M. Solomon, Displacement of Drugs from Plasma Binding Sites as a Factor in Drug Toxicity. In S. W. Goldstein (Ed.), *Safer and More Effective Drugs*. Courtesy of The American Pharmaceutical Association-Academy of Pharmaceutical Sciences, Washington, D.C.

Simultaneously, the antidiabetic agent is metabolized slower than usual, and there is an increase in the hypoglycemic effect.

DRUG INTERACTIONS AT THE RECEPTOR SITE

A basic concept of drug action is that the pharmacologic action of a compound is ultimately due to the drug's adsorption onto a receptor site. Drug interactions can occur when a drug that does not give a response occupies the receptor sites normally used by an active drug. Examples are shown in Table 6-II, where an antagonist drug crowds out an agonist drug; the normal function of the agonist is prevented. Amphetamines and tricyclic antidepressant drugs can interfere with the action of guanethedine, an antihypertensive drug. The result is an increase in blood pressure. A patient taking pilocarpine drops for glaucoma may notice a decrease in activity if antispasmodic drugs (anticholinergics) were prescribed for ulcers or some other gastrointestinal disorder.

TABLE 6-II
INTERACTIONS AT THE RECEPTOR SITE

Antagonist Drug	Agonist Drug
Atropine	Acetylcholine
Gallamine (Flaxedil®)	Succinylcholine (Anectine®)
Amphetamine and methylphenidate	Guanethidine (Ismelin)
Imipramine (Tofranil) and other tricyclic antidepressants	Guanethidine (Ismelin)
Propranolol (Inderal®)	Isoproterenol (Isuprel®, Norisodrine®)
Anticholinergics (atropine, Banthine®, Pro-Banthine®, etc.)	Pilocarpine

DRUG INTERACTIONS ASSOCIATED WITH RENAL EXCRETION

Most drugs are excreted largely by the kidneys, either as the free drug or as water-soluble metabolites, and urinary pH (acidity or alkalinity) can influence the activity of a drug by altering the rate of renal clearance. However, alteration of urinary pH by drugs such as sodium bicarbonate or ammonium chloride is a rare occurrence, and unless the pH change is sustained for a relatively long period of time, there is probably no clinically significant result.

Urinary pH can influence antimicrobial therapy of urinary tract infections. Methenamine, tetracyclines, and nitrofurantoins are most active when the urine is acidic (pH is 5.5 or less). Patients taking these drugs for urinary tract infections should be encouraged to drink plenty of fluids, including cranberry juice.

Renal function is one of the most important factors determining drug activity. If a drug is primarily excreted by the kidneys in an unchanged form, it is important that the patient's renal status is known. Adverse drug reactions in patients with impaired renal function have been reported to be two and one-half times those of patients with normal renal function.[4] When renal function is impaired, the rate of excretion of a drug normally excreted by the kidneys is slowed down. As additional doses of the drug are taken, the blood levels build up, possibly to a toxic level. Therefore, the doses of drugs such as digitalis and gentamycin should be adjusted downward in patients with reduced renal function.

Some drugs may compete for specialized excretion sites in the kidneys. For example, furosemide (Lasix®), a potent diuretic, competes with salicylate excretion in the kidney tubules, and salicylate toxicity may result.

OTHER TYPES OF DRUG INTERACTION

There are several other important drug-drug interactions that may contribute to dangerous increases in drug activity. The concurrent or sequential administration of two or more agents possessing similar pharmacologic actions or side effects may give rise to drug interactions by the additive or synergistic effect of these properties. The more obvious examples are the administration of central nervous system (CNS) depressants (barbiturates, tranquilizers, narcotic analgesics) with each other. Serious motor and mental impairments can occur when these drugs are taken together. Another important problem is the drug-drug interaction associated with the ingestion of CNS depressants along with alcoholic beverages.

The administration of one drug with the potential to alter the basic mechanism of another drug can also result in a drug interaction. The interaction is not a simple additive effect but is a result of drug-induced changes in the patient. For example, thiazide diuretics (Esidrix®, HydroDIURIL), by producing potassium (an electrolyte that influences electrical signals in the heart) loss via urinary excretion can predispose patients to toxic reactions from cardiac glycosides such as digitalis. Potassium-containing foods (beef, orange juice, bananas) and supplements should be an important part of the patient's regimen when taking these drugs.

STRATEGY FOR MINIMIZING DRUG INTERACTIONS

In the light of the foregoing information on potential drug interactions among elderly patients, there are a number of specific actions that should be taken to help minimize the likelihood and danger of such interactions. Although these actions should be viewed as routine, they should be only part of a comprehensive medical and pharmaceutical strategy for the prevention of all types of drug-related problems to which older patients are subject.

1. Awareness—The key to preventing a drug interaction is keeping the possibility of such an occurrence in mind whenever dealing with an elderly patient who is likely to be taking more than one drug. This is especially important with patients being treated for hypertension or cardiovascular conditions or those who have liver and renal diseases.
2. Maintain patient medical history and drug profile—Records of all drugs (both prescription and over-the-counter) used by the patient should be maintained by physicians, pharmacies, nursing homes, and other extended-care facilities. Records should also be kept on the patient's general medical condition and any history of adverse drug reactions. These records serve as a good reference point for detecting potential drug interaction problems or for diagnosing already-existing adverse reactions in patients.
3. Careful monitoring of patient—The practitioner should watch carefully for unusual changes in the condition or behavior of patients taking more than one drug, patients switched from one drug to another, or patients taken off one or more drugs and maintained on others.

REFERENCES

1. Doluisio, J. T., La Piana, J. C., Wilkinson, G. R., and Dittert, L. W.: Pharmacokinetic interpretation of dicloxacillin levels in serum after extravascular administration. In Hobby, G . L. (Ed.): *Antimicrobial Agents and Chemotherapy—1969.* Bethesda, Maryland, American Society for Microbiology, 1970.
2. Melmon, K. L.: Preventable drug reactions—Causes and cures. *N Engl J Med, 284*:1361-1367, 1971.
3. Scheiner, J. and Altemeier, W. A.: Experimental study of factors inhibiting absorption and effective therapeutic levels of declomycin. *Surg Gynecol Obstet, 114*:9-14, 1962.

4. Smith, J. W., Seidl, L. G., and Cluff, L. E.: Studies on the epidemiology of adverse drug reactions. *Ann Intern Med, 65*:629-640, 1966.
5. Solomon, H. M.: Displacement of drugs from plasma binding sites as a factor in drug toxicity. In Goldstein, S. W. (Ed.): *Safer and More Effective Drugs.* Washington, D.C., American Pharmaceutical Association, Academy of Pharmaceutical Sciences, 1968.
6. Wagner, J. G.: Design and analysis of biopharmaceutical studies in man. *Can J Pharm Sci, 1*:55-68, 1966.

Chapter 7

PHARMACEUTICAL SERVICES FOR THE ELDERLY PATIENT

ALBERT W. JOWDY, PH.D.
CHARLES L. BRAUCHER, PH.D.

IN ANY DISCUSSION of the pharmaceutical services for the elderly, it is essential that the drug *needs* of the elderly be considered. Drug needs are directly related to the state of health of the individual. In a sense, then, drug needs are health needs.

An assessment of pharmaceutical services for the elderly must also include an analysis of the health and drug needs expressed by the elderly themselves, as well as a perception of those needs by the pharmaceutical and medical professions. This is because the elderly have relatively easy access to drugs through either self-medication with nonprescription drugs or professionally controlled medication with drugs restricted to prescription.

In a study of the status and needs of the older person in relatively rural communities, Belcher and Deutschberger reported on the response of 1,154 persons above the age of sixty-five who were asked to classify their health status. Three percent evaluated their health as excellent, 18 percent listed good health, 47 percent said they were in fair health, and 32 percent considered themselves in poor health. From the data presented, the investigators concluded that "it is obvious that the individual's assessment of his health is very much related to the problems he feels confront him and to his general perception of life."[1]

In another study, 895 Georgia citizens over sixty-five years of age were interviewed to determine their actual social conditions. Among the social indicators reported was "self-expressed need for service." The report of this study noted that 80 percent of the persons aged sixty-five and over appear to be self-sufficient and the remaining 20 percent not self-sufficient. The most frequent requests for help were voiced by those people who were interested in "getting better medical care" (35 percent). Persons living in rural areas were found to have more requests for help in meeting what they perceived as their needs than those who lived in urban areas.[13]

The health and drug needs of the elderly as seen by the medical and pharmaceutical professionals may differ somewhat from the elderly's own perception of their needs. In any society, there are many problems which all members, including the aged, must face. But to the aged, illness may be seen as a catastrophe that can reduce or remove their independence.

Those in the health care field may view the health needs of the elderly as having parameters including more than the medical problem alone. This outlook was stated by Devas[5] in discussing problems associated with the practice of geriatric medicine:

> The principles of geriatric medicine and surgery are the same as at any other age but they have to be applied with the utmost vigor from the moment of admission to ultimate discharge from outpatients (so-called "total care"). The circumstances in which the patients live, financial problems, the surgical condition, the concomitant medical afflictions, how rehabilitation and the social services can best be used, nursing care and, most important, the morale of the patient, all have to be carefully considered. It must be remembered that in the elderly loss of function means loss of independence.[5]

In addition to these considerations, there are personality strains which may reflect the psychological and physical factors involved in the aging process. This consideration was emphasized by Stanaszek:

> There are several psychological factors inherent in the "stress of aging" such as retirement, lowered social status, role reversal, loss by death of friends and relatives, and decrease in intellectual capacity. Decreased physical abilities manifest themselves in the form of: (a) slowing down of all body systems and physical functioning; (b) increased incidence of illness; (c) slower rate of recovery; (d) greater possibility of residual impairment. Personalities of geriatric patients often reflect many of the factors mentioned above.[16]

DRUG NEEDS OF THE ELDERLY

Chen, in discussing pharmacological factors in geriatrics, stressed the importance of prophylactic measures for the elderly. He argued that persons should be educated to recognize and understand the normal aging process long before they approach old age. Drugs, he noted, could not be used to retard or reverse that process but only to diminish the impact of disease and ease some of the associated discomforts.[2]

In the selection of drugs for use by elderly patients, knowledge of the drug must be considered along with those age-related changes that might be favorably or adversely influenced. Moreover, drugs have become more plentiful, and the indications for their use have become more specific. Therefore, as increasingly specific medications are developed, there is less room for deviations from clearly stated pharmacological principles in treatment of the elderly patient.[6]

A major consideration in assessing the drug needs of geriatric patients is their physiological ability to handle drugs. As Hall has noted, ". . . the elderly differ from younger people in their response to drugs, for their ability to handle drugs by absorption, detoxication, and excretion is naturally affected. Not surprisingly, therefore, iatrogenic diesase related to drugs is very common."[7]

Another problem concerning the drug needs of the elderly is the very real possibility of multiple disease conditions existing concurrently in the same patient. Multiple morbidity is not only common in the elderly patient but is further complicated by the fact that some diseases require more than one drug. Therefore, if every complaint were treated, the result could be dangerous polypharmacy, or regimens of self-defeating complexity.[4]

The drug needs of the elderly have been systematized by Wenzel, who listed six general principles for geriatric drug therapy:

(1) The pattern of living should not be markedly changed by the use of drugs. Activity patterns, sleeping and eating times, etc. should be disturbed as little as possible.
(2) Treatment details, especially for the self-administration of medication, should be as simple as possible. Complex dosage patterns with multiple drugs can lead to confusion and over- or under-

dosage. Liquid preparations that must be carefully measured, e.g. tincture of digitalis or tincture of belladonna, can be dangerous.
(3) Established drug habits with real or placebo effects, if changed or broken, must be handled with care. Cathartics, aspirin, vitamins, antacids, etc. when withdrawn may produce direct or psychologically-induced symptoms.
(4) As most geriatric therapy is chronic, drug selection must include consideration of cumulative toxicity, addiction, tolerance, and cost.
(5) Because the aging human responds differently to many drugs than his youthful counterpart, specific differences should be understood.
(6) As the usual senior citizen has limited purchasing power, the cost/effectiveness ratio becomes of considerable importance. An expensive drug that a person will not purchase is of no therapeutic value.[19]

TYPES OF DRUG PROBLEMS AMONG THE ELDERLY

Self-medication by the elderly raises the possibility of medication misuse. One study of the misuse of prescription medications by outpatients, conducted by Latiolais and Berry, found that the older patient is more likely to misuse his medication.[10] Another study by Malahy attempted to find a relationship between age, education, number of medications taken, and medication errors. The results showed that there was no relationship between the patient's age or education and the number of medication errors made. This investigation did, however, find that the number of medications taken by the patient was the only variable related to medication errors.[12]

The connection between age and frequency of drug use led Rabin to comment, "As one would expect from their greater morbidity, older persons acquire and use more prescribed medicines than do younger persons. Advancing age consistently predicted increased prescribed drug use. . . ."[14] Since the elderly take more medications, it is reasonable to assume that medication errors would increase proportionately. This relationship, however, may not always hold.[14]

Schwartz and her associates[15] found that finer age-groupings produce a clouded picture of the relationship between medication errors and age. Using five-year intervals for people age sixty and over, these investigators found the proportion of error makers for each group to be: age 60-64 (55%); 65-69 (65%); 70-74 (51%); 75-79 (80%); 80-84 (70%); 85 and over (25%). The authors concluded, "That the oldest patients were least likely to make errors is somewhat surprising, and may in part be a result of the very small number of patients (eight) in this group. Nevertheless, one may speculate that relatives, physicians, visiting nurses, and neighbors tend to be more protective of the very old."[15]

The same investigators found that the types of medication errors made by the elderly were, in rank order, the following: omission of medication, 47 percent; inaccurate knowledge, 20 percent; self-medication, 17 percent; incorrect dosage, 10 percent; and improper timing or sequence, 6 percent. In commenting on this finding, the researchers stated that problems of communication between professional personnel and patient are clearly involved in medication errors due to inaccurate knowledge. In regard to self-medication errors, slightly over one-third of all error makers were found to be taking one or more medications not ordered by the physician. Patients' comments regarding dosage sequence and timing errors suggest that at least some of the errors may be accounted for by poor eyesight and confusion about which instructions belong with which medication.[15]

The potential for harm to the elderly through medication errors appears even greater in the light of one study which found that 5 percent of the patients admitted to a hospital had a drug-induced disease on admission.[17] The serious nature of the problems created by self-medication among the elderly is further emphasized by the fact that, even under the controlled conditions of a hospital, an estimated 18 to 30 percent of all hospitalized patients experience a drug reaction while hospitalized and that the duration of their hospital stay is nearly doubled as a result.[9]

The possibility of an elderly patient "shopping around" for physicians can also produce problems which should properly be classified as medication duplication rather than error. One physician associated with the Kansas University Medical Center reported as follows:

> Many elderly patients don't really stick with one physician. . . . They visit a private practitioner in town frequently, and occasionally

they drop into the K.U. Medical Center and sometimes over to General Hospital. I've seen patients that are taking 18 different kinds of medicine every day. I've seen patients taking 3 different kinds of digitalis preparations prescribed by different doctors. Now, maybe the doctor goofed or his records were bad or maybe he forgot like all of us do. That's inexcusable. But most of the time, it really wasn't the physician's error at all. Most of the time it's because the patient was doing a little doctor shopping. The only person who might be in a position to pick up this kind of thing is the neighborhood pharmacist.[8]

In addition to the possibility of medication error or duplication, the elderly patient is faced with a far more complex threat to his or her health security—drug reactions and/or drug interactions. As Hussar has mentioned, "When considering the risk of drug reactions, age is a particularly important factor. Studies indicate that there is an increased incidence of adverse drug reactions in pediatric and geriatric patients, and one estimate suggests that the risk of a drug reaction in patients 60-70 years of age is almost double that in adults 30-40 years old."[9]

In discussing the pharmacological considerations in aging, Leake points out the dangers inherent in drug reactions due to physiological changes in the elderly.

> In adapting pharmacological principles to the aging, there is one obligatory proposition: Drugs can only make living cells do more or less what they are already capable of doing. If the cells are depleted, or if the tissues are senescent, drugs are limited. . . .
> Drugs in older individuals are subject to new considerations in terms of reactive time and reactive capacity. Synergism and imbalances due to the interaction of compounds are more likely to cause immediate drastic results as well as long-term undue effects. Medications in older people tend to produce irreversible effects in tissues as well as in functions. Compensable capacities are constricted. For example, hypotension inadvertently induced by drugs in a younger person is not as hazardous as in an older person in whom cerebral symptoms are more likely to occur earlier and with greater intensity. Effects of epinephrine in the younger person may be transient and relatively inconsequential whereas the drug can induce irremediable changes in the cardiovascular, renal, and cerebral circulation in the old.[11]

In addition to the above drug reactions, the health of the elderly can also be threatened by drug interactions, a phenomenon which has been defined as "those situations where the effects of one drug are altered by the prior or concurrent administration of another."[9]

PHARMACEUTICAL SERVICES FOR THE ELDERLY PATIENT

Pharmaceutical services for the elderly are a necessity if the serious problems of medication errors, drug duplication, physician shopping, drug reactions, and drug interactions are to be reduced or, hopefully, eliminated. This can come about by firmly establishing control of medication by the pharmacist as a means of monitoring drug usage by the elderly. Such drug monitoring is important for both the institutionalized patient and the noninstitutionalized patient.

The institutionalized elderly patient now has, or can have in the future, the benefit of clinical pharmacy services designed to prevent those problems surrounding drug usage by the elderly which have been the subject of this discussion. The federal Task Force on the Pharmacist's Clinical Role[18] has recommended that hospitals, extended care facilities, and nursing homes institute clinical pharmacy services, such as dispensing and administering drugs, document professional activities, direct patient involvement, and review of drug utilization, education, and consultation. Many of these services are already available for institutionalized patients.

The noninstitutionalized elderly patient has daily access to the pharmacist in a community pharmacy or in an outpatient health care center. Financial coverage for drugs through Medicaid, Medicare, and private health insurance arrangements has increased the number of elderly patients who are having prescriptions filled in noninstitutional pharmacies. From this consideration, it follows that pharmacists will have increasing opportunities to serve the elderly patient.

The community pharmacist is able to serve elderly patients in many ways. For example, he is available for consultation on prescription and nonprescription medication; he provides written and verbal instructions for the proper use and storage of drugs; he suggests the availability and use of prescription and sickroom accessory items; he assists in organizing medication schedules; and he may maintain a patient profile system to prevent drug interactions or adverse drug effects. The pharmacist may also counsel elderly patients on the importance of following the prescribed drug therapy program, because some patients may have negative attitudes regarding drug use. Such attitudes may originate from ethnic or religious backgrounds that hinder full compliance with therapy.[16]

The noninstitutionalized elderly patient can also benefit from personal medication monitoring conducted by the community pharmacist. This usually consists of two types: (1) medication calendars and (2) patient or family medication records. Medication calendars assist in determining renewal dates for patients on maintenance medication. By consulting the medication calendar, the pharmacist can prepare the patient's medication in advance so that it is ready when reordered by the patient. The calendar may also be used to indicate the extent to which the patient is still taking medication according to the physician's instructions.

Closely related to the medication calendar is the activity involved in planning a medication schedule. Stanaszek has pointed out the rationale for this service: "Elderly persons often take many medications, and need assistance in developing a schedule for correct use of these medications.... The pharmacist can provide a great professional service in this area by planning an individual medication schedule program for the geriatric patient. Correlating medication schedules with meals or bedtime, whenever possible, may significantly increase patient compliance with drug orders."[16] Patient or family medication records generally are kept for the protection of the patient as a service of the community pharmacy. Close and Danian have listed some of the most important reasons for using patient, or family, medication records in the community pharmacy.

(1) The potential danger to the patient who sees more than one physician, each of whom may be unfamiliar with the patient's drug regimen;
(2) The possibility of harm to the patient taking drugs that interact with certain disease states or allergies;
(3) The potential for harm to the patient due to drug interactions

involving o-t-c [over-the-counter] drugs with legend drugs and interactions of legend drugs with one another;

(4) The providing of information which is needed by a patient who has changed his physician or moved to another community and has lost his prescription container.[3]

Patient record systems vary from community pharmacy to community pharmacy; however, there are several major information entries which would probably be common to most systems. Recorded information may include the following: patient's name, sex, date of birth, Social Security number, address, telephone number, names of family members, emergency contact, weight, allergies, sensitivities, reactions, chronic disease conditions, prescription number, product name (manufacturer), date drug dispensed, strength, quantity, refills authorized, date of refills, dosage form, directions for use, and the prescriber's name.[3]

Considering the possibilities of medication error, drug-drug interactions, drug-food interactions, unreported use of nonprescription drugs, allergies, drug sensitivities, and age-associated physical impairments, medication record systems are a necessity to adequately protect the health and well-being of the elderly patient who is using medication. The professional pharmacist is able to provide those pharmaceutical services necessary to facilitate this protection.

CONCLUSION

Pharmaceutical services for the elderly are a necessity if the serious problems of medication errors, drug duplication, physician shopping, drug reactions, and drug interactions are to be reduced or eliminated. These problems of the elderly patient can eventually be solved by the provision of adequate clinical pharmacy services for the institutionalized patient and personal medication monitoring by the community pharmacist for the noninstitutionalized patient. Through the use of medication calendars and patient, or family, medication records, the community pharmacist can exercise some control over the drug-usage pattern of the elderly. Through professional consultation with both the patient and his physician, the pharmacist, in the institution and the community, can provide the catalyst for the rational use of drugs in the management of the elderly patient.

REFERENCES

1. Belcher, J. C. and Deutschberger, S.: *Needs of Older Persons in Nonmetropolitan Communities.* Report of the University of Georgia School of Social Work and the Athens Chapter of the Georgia Gerontology Society, Inc., Athens, Georgia, The Northeast Georgia Area Planning and Development Commission, 1966.
2. Chen, K. K.: Principles of pharmacology as applied to the aged. In Stieglitz, E. J. (Ed.): *Geriatric Medicine.* Philadelphia, Saunders, 1943.
3. Close, C. and Danian, M.: The value of the use of the family medication record. *J Am Pharm Assoc, NS13*:342-344, 1973.
4. Currie, G., MacNeill, R. M., Walker, T. G., and Mudie, E. W.: Medical and social screening of patients aged 70 to 72, by an urban general practice health team. *Br Med J, 2*:108-111, 1974.
5. Devas, M. B.: Geriatric orthopedics. *Br Med J, 1*:190-192, 1974.
6. Freeman, J. T.: General introduction. In Freeman, J. T. (Ed.): *Clinical Principles and Drugs in the Aging.* Springfield, Thomas, 1963.
7. Hall, M. R. P.: Drug therapy in the elderly. *Br Med J, 4*:582-584, 1973.
8. Hastings, G.: Concepts in geriatric treatment. *Seminar Proceedings: Short-Term Training Program For Medical Care Facility Nurses and the Pharmacist Consultant.* Kansas City, University of Missouri Division for Continuing Education, 1967.
9. Hussar, D. A.: Drug interactions—Introduction and general principles. *Conn Pharmacist, 34*:9-12, 1972.
10. Latiolais, C. J. and Berry, C. C.: Misuse of prescription medications by outpatients. *Drug Intell Clin Pharm, 3*:270-277, 1969.
11. Leake, C. D.: Principles and practices in the geriatric use of drugs. In Freeman, J. T. (Ed.): *Clinical Principles and Drugs in the Aging.* Springfield, Thomas, 1963.
12. Malahy, B.: The effect of instruction and labeling on the number of medication errors made by patients at home. *Am J Hosp Pharm, 23*:283-292, 1966.
13. Office of Aging: *Social Indicators for the Aged.* Atlanta, Georgia Department of Human Resources, 1972.
14. Rabin, D. L.: Use of medicine: A review of prescribed and nonprescribed medicine use. *Reprint Series*: 668-699, Washington, D.C., U.S. Department of Health, Education and Welfare, 1972.
15. Schwartz, D., Wang, M., Zeitz, L., and Goss, M. E. W.: Medication errors made by elderly chronically ill patients. *Am J Public Health, 52*:2018-2029, 1962.
16. Stanaszek, W. F.: How pharmacists can serve geriatric patients more effectively. *Pharm Times, 40*:28-33, 1974.

17. Stewart, R. B. and Cluff, L. E.: A review of medication errors and compliance in ambulant patients. *Clin Pharmacol Ther, 13*:463-468, 1972.
18. Task Force on the Pharmacist's Clinical Role: *National Center for Health Services Research and Development Briefs, Report No. 4.* Washington, D.C., Department of Health, Education and Welfare, 1971.
19. Wenzel, D.: Drugs and the aging population. *Seminar Proceedings: Short-Term Training Program For Medical Care Facility Nurses and the Pharmacist Consultant.* Kansas City, University of Missouri Division for Continuing Education, 1967.

Chapter 8

SELF-MEDICATION PROBLEMS AMONG THE ELDERLY*

FLYNN WARREN, M.S.

SELF-MEDICATION IS A reality today no matter which meaning of the term is under discussion. *Self-medication* has been used to describe either of two actions: (1) the self-treatment of some medical problem using medications that were not obtained by a visit to a physician concerned with the problem or (2) the self-administration of medications prescribed for a patient by a physician. In this chapter, the term *self-medication* is largely employed to discuss the use of over-the-counter or nonprescription medications to treat problems that the patient does not deem serious enough to require the attention of a physician.[2] Similarly, *self-administration* is used to refer to a patient taking prescribed medications as part of a total plan of treatment for some condition. The compliance of the patient with the prescribed regimen is the most common framework for the discussion of self-administration of drugs.[20] Both definitions are discussed in this chapter.

SELF-MEDICATION

Why do people self-medicate rather than visit a physician? Among the most commonly cited reasons for self-medication is the inability to see a physician when needed. Other reasons include the lack of money to pay the physician for writing a prescription and, related to this, the tendency to treat oneself for the limited, minor medical conditions that go away anyway if only endured for a few days. The self-medication, in this

---

* Many of the issues discussed in this chapter, while relevant to the elderly, are also germane to the nonelderly.

instance, is used for the temporary alleviation of symptoms associated with the condition present. Examples of such conditions include the common cold, slight nausea, occasional diarrhea or constipation, coughs, transient headaches, and minor cuts.

The problems of not being able to see a physician and the cost of treatment can be very real. Patients express extreme dislike of the waiting time in hospital emergency rooms—despite this, there is acknowledged misuse of emergency facilities and personnel. Also, with the number and type of medical specialists in practice today, getting to see the right physician can also be a problem. Even when a physician is available, the patient may be reluctant to use a visit to the physician's office for the treatment of a seemingly minor condition. In this instance, cost is the predominant factor. In addition to the actual fee charged by the physician, many patients must contend with loss of income due to absence from their job, the problem of transportation to the physician's office, and the cost of an expensive prescription medication. To patients on limited income (which includes most of the elderly), such financial problems may outweigh the desire for proper, full medical attention. As an alternative to the physician visit, the local pharmacy is open, no appointment is needed, and the drugs can be purchased there. In summary, the use of self-medication, under the proper circumstances, can be a quick, inexpensive source of drug therapy.

One problem pervades the entire spectrum of self-medication, however. This is the ability of the patient to select the proper treatment for the condition from which the patient is suffering. That is, how accurately can a nonphysician "diagnose" the problems present and arrive at the proper choice of drug therapy? Obviously there are many difficulties involved in a lay person arriving at the proper decision. The result is that the self-medicating patient usually treats a symptom rather than attempting to treat the specific medical condition that is present. An example of such symptomatic therapy would be the likely treatment for a toothache. The basic pathological condition present, for example, is a cavity in the involved tooth, but the patient's sensation is that of pain in the area. The remedy desired is some form of either systemic or local analgesic. The analgesic preparation probably relieves the pain, but the real disease process, the cavity, remains unaltered. The drug therapy employed in this case has worked to bring about relief of the problem bothering the patient.

The natural extension of the ability of the patient to use drugs, through self-medication, to relieve symptoms of disease is the danger that the use of self-medication, on a prolonged basis, permits the user to avoid seeking needed medical treatment. Such fears are based on solid evidence when one considers the almost bizarre patterns of medication use that patients can develop.[7] In a similar fashion, the continued use of over-the-counter medications by a patient could confuse the physician's diagnostic evaluation of the patient's medical problem. Such potential problems must be acknowledged and guarded against in patients who are known to employ self-medication on a regular or chronic basis. The complete medication history, whether taken by a physician or pharmacist, must include information and questions relating the patient's use of nonprescription drugs to the complaints from which the patient suffers. It has often been mentioned in studies performed on patients and their drug histories that many patients do not mention commonly taken drugs such as aspirin and laxatives during questioning unless they are specifically asked about the use of these agents.[18, 22]

Another problem that must be kept in mind with patients that are using self-medication is the potential for drug interactions that exists. The subject of drug interactions is dealt with as a distinct subject in Chapter 6 and is not duplicated here. Further, a voluminous amount of literature exists on the subject, and the reader can readily satisfy his need for information on this topic. The Food and Drug Administration is undertaking, as a component of its review of all over-the-counter drug products, to ensure that adequate labeling is provided to caution the patient concerning the improper use of these medications, including drug interactions.[27]

Once the decision has been made by the patient to employ an over-the-counter drug for self-medication, what forces come to bear to influence the choice of the specific product that will be purchased? The most dominant factor, when operating, is previous experience with the drug product being considered. This experience may have been either positive (it worked before) or negative (it did not perform satisfactorily before). In the latter case, the patient is now shopping for a different drug product to use. Drug products that have performed well during previous uses are likely to be selected for future use when a product of that class is needed.

The recommendations of friends constitute a form of persuasive advertising in the selection of many items, and over-the-counter drugs are no exception. If the problem to be treated is discussed with a friend of the patient, it may be that the friend has personally used a needed drug product previously and can attest to its effectiveness or ineffectiveness as appropriate. Every pharmacist could cite, however, numerous episodes when persons come into the pharmacy seeking a product and possess only a "sounds-like" or "used-for" piece of information about the drug product. The failure to get the information correctly from friends can have dire consequences if the wrong product is purchased.[28]

The advertising of over-the-counter medications in every available media form has been the subject of great controversy with positions being taken that advertising of nonprescription medications both does[14] and does not[15] increase the use of such agents. The actual fact probably lies somewhere between the two extremes. Although the Food and Drug Administration has control over the marketing and the labeling of all nonprescription medications, the advertising of the products is controlled by the Federal Trade Commission. The limitations on labeling, as imposed by the Food and Drug Administration, guide the Federal Trade Commission in its decisions of what is fair to advertise about the benefits of a particular drug product and what can be considered to be beyond the limits of claims for a given product. Two excellent reviews of this relationship have appeared in the recent literature.[6, 12]

In addition to advertising within the media, the level of advertisement given the product within the particular store the patient uses can influence whether or not a particular product is purchased. Any drug product may be prominently displayed on any given day in such a manner to attract the attention of potential purchasers. Products that are hidden by their placement in the store are not likely to be selected as a spontaneous purchase by the customer. The appeal of the package itself, almost without regard to the product within, can also be a source of purchase initiation. Arrangement of related items on the shelves can also stimulate the purchase of one brand rather than another in some circumstances. For example, the brand of antibacterial ointment displayed with the bandage section is more likely to be purchased than the one three aisles away. While all of the considerations above have a scientific basis from a marketing standpoint, they usually have little, if any, scientific rationale from a therapeutics standpoint.

Price of a product is always going to have an influence on whether or not it is selected for purchase and especially when two similar items can be compared by price alone. In many cases, sale items are the popular choice simply because they are on sale. Many of the same arguments that have been advanced concerning the duplicity of the pricing structure for packaged foods could be made about packaged drugs for over-the-counter sale. The same pressures that have given rise to unit pricing in supermarkets for food items could be applied to the pricing of over-the-counter drugs. The definition of the unit that will serve as the basis for drug pricing may be more difficult to establish, however, than is the decision to price all cereal products on the basis of per ounce of cereal. It might seem easy to say that the price should be per ounce of liquid medications and per tablet or capsule for the oral solid medications. Such a price-comparison method could be confusing and inaccurate when the dosage of the two products was different.

We might consider, for example, the comparison pricing between two liquid vitamin-mineral supplements designed to be taken once a day as a source of additional vitamins and iron. Product A is supplied in 12-ounce bottles at a price of $3.60 per bottle. The competition, Product B, is available in 8-ounce bottles that cost $4.80 each. On immediate examination, the choice of Product A at a cost of thirty cents an ounce seems preferable to the purchase of Product B at a price of sixty cents an ounce, if price alone is the determinant for selection. However, careful reading of the label, with regard to drug content of the preparations and recommended dosage, reveals that the patient must take 1 ounce (30 ml or 2 tablespoonsful) of Product A to get the same quantity of active ingredients present in 5 ml (1 teaspoonful) of Product B. The true price comparison, then, using per dose as the basis, becomes thirty cents for a 30 ml dose of Product A, but only ten cents for the 5 ml dose of Product B. Thus, even though the actual purchase price is higher and the bottle purchased is smaller, Product B is a better buy for the cost-conscious consumer. Similar illustrations could be given for many drug products. Asking the pharmacist for such comparisons is a wise decision when purchasing over-the-counter drug products.

The advice of the pharmacist is often sought for the purchase of an over-the-counter drug product when the purchaser has no idea what the most appropriate product would be. It should be emphasized at this point that pharmacists are not trained in the art and science of physical diagnosis as a regular part of their formal education. Hence, a pharmacist is neither legally nor illegally able to accurately diagnose the medical condition with which a patient may present. A fair assessment of the role that a pharmacist can play in the "diagnosis" of the patient's problem is to caution the patient in the use of certain medications that would be contraindicated in certain circumstances. Perhaps the most important role that the pharmacist has in the recommendation of over-the-counter products is in knowing when not to sell a product to the customer. In this case, the patient comes into the pharmacy and asks for assistance in the selection of a treatment for a given condition. If self-medication is inappropriate, the pharmacist tells this to the patient and also states why it is inappropriate for the patient at this time. The proper method of treatment may be referral of the patient to a physician in order that a correct medical treatment can be begun. The role of the pharmacist may evolve to that of a modified triage officer in aiding patients in obtaining the correct form of medical care.

What are some of the other advantages to the patient who chooses to employ self-medication in the treatment of minor conditions? While many older over-the-counter drug products often sought to conceal their contents through improper labels, the new regulations relating to the labeling and sale of over-the-counter medications insure that accurate, factual information is

Self-Medication Problems Among the Elderly

available to the purchaser. This information includes directions for proper use, conditions under which use of the drug is not indicated, conditions which might be masked by using the drug, dosage that is appropriate, and side effects that might occur. Additional information on storage of the drug and any needed information appropriate to each particular drug may also be provided. It should be remembered, however, that all the labeling in the world is useless if unheeded.[26] Some sound professional advice to the patient is always valuable.

An additional advantage of over-the-counter medications is the ability of the patient to purchase effective drugs without a prescription. Most lay persons probably harbor a great deal of doubt about the efficacy or potency of nonprescription drugs. This is a needless worry. One of the considerations of the Food and Drug Administration review of the ingredients of over-the-counter products is that they are present in quantities sufficient to be effective as well as safe. Further, many drugs that are thought of as prescription drugs may actually be sold without a prescription. Many of the over-the-counter cold preparations are simply the prescription-only version in different packaging. This is also true for cough syrups and many topical preparations. Thus, the patient who selects an over-the-counter remedy can be relatively certain that the product purchased contains only ingredients that are effective, present in proper quantities, and labeled for proper and effective use.

Another advantage of using an over-the-counter drug, especially when compared to some of the other self-medication treatment possibilities to be discussed, is the willingness of the patient to admit its use when questioned by a physician. In this case, the over-the-counter drug has been used for a limited time, the patient's symptoms have not improved, and the patient has then decided to visit a physician. Human nature being what it is, the patient is probably more likely to admit the use of a "legitimate" drug source to the physician than in the case of other possible drug sources, which will be discussed.

Self-medication can also be accomplished with prescription medications, and two methods of obtaining prescription drugs without proper medical supervision can be considered. The first method is the exchange of prescription drugs between friends, and the second is the use of drugs previously prescribed for the patient by a physician. Each of these is considered separately, for each has its own special set of problems and benefits.

How can one obtain prescription drugs other than by going to a physician? One method is to request the drug from a friend known to possess the desired drug. Second, a friend may also simply volunteer to provide the medication when the problem is discussed jointly. Third, the drug may be obtained from a member of the health community who has access to the drug from some legitimate source of supply and who takes it by theft or similar means. Examples of the third method include the pharmacist who yields to pressure from a good friend and sells the drug without a prescription, the physician's office personnel who obtain samples for friends to use, hospital employees who expropriate medications issued to them for patients' use as needed on outings away from the hospital, and even the physician who issues prescriptions to friends and family members without first determining the need for such medications.

Improperly obtained medications are usually quickly available, unless there is some delay when they must be "obtained" from sources that would not normally provide the drugs without question. They usually also are available for little or no cost, and this makes their use attractive. The patient is assured of the use of a potent drug product for treatment of his condition and can, therefore, feel that this method is superior to the use of a nonprescription drug. All these are considered to be advantages to the use of such drugs.

The disadvantages of using improperly obtained prescription drugs can be important. The difficulty the patient has in accurately assessing the nature and severity of his condition is still inherent in this method. The likelihood of the patient experiencing a serious side effect from the use of the drug is probably greater when using a prescription drug than is the case when using a nonprescription drug. This side effect could be serious in nature and many require the patient to seek medical assistance for treatment of the side effect alone. If the chosen drug therapy fails to work, and the patient must then seek the advice of a physician, he or she may be quite reluctant to admit the use of such a medication to the physician. Absence of this knowledge could hamper the physician in his assessment of the patient's condition. Anytime a patient is using a prescription drug that is in an improperly labeled container, which would be any drug that has not been labeled as a prescription drug by a pharmacist, there is the possibility of misinterpretation of directions given with the drug by the provider. As will be shown later, patients can often misinterpret the directions for taking a medication even when the container is clearly labeled. The unlabeled bottle of medication is a greater invitation for drug-administration error. A second danger for using improperly labeled medications can occur if the drug in question is a controlled substance.* A person in possession of a controlled substance, obtained without a prescription, might be charged with either a misdemeanor or felony violation, depending on the circumstances of the occurrence and the laws of the locality in which the event took place.

The other potential circumstance for the use of a prescription drug in the self-medication of patients is for the patient to reuse a drug product that has been previously prescribed for the same or a similar condition. Such drugs may already be on hand in the home or can be obtained by the refilling of an open prescription at the pharmacy. This form of prescription drug use does have the advantage of the drug having previously been matched to the patient by a physician, and this decreases the likelihood of an allergic or serious adverse reaction to the drug product. Also, the same set of symptoms that are presently concerning the patient had been previously diagnosed by the physician who prescribed the drug originally. These factors work to the patient's advantage to increase the likelihood of the self-medication being successful.

Other advantages of reuse of a previously prescribed medication include the ready availability of the medication with only a trip to the neighborhood pharmacy as a likely delay. If the medication is already on hand, there is no cost and, even if the

---

* A controlled substance is a drug entity that is subject to abuse. This includes narcotics, amphetamines, barbiturates, sedatives, and some of the minor tranquilizers. Federal, state, and local governmental laws concern their distribution, and transfer between patients is expressly forbidden by federal regulation.

prescription must be refilled, the cost is still relatively low for most drugs. The patient does have the use of a potent drug once more, but the safety factor is better when using a drug that was originally obtained by prescription than when using one obtained without a physician visit.

One peculiar disadvantage to the reuse method may lie in the fact that the drug product has been stored since it was originally dispensed by the pharmacy, and the patient may not have kept the drug under the proper conditions to prevent its deterioration. The product may also simply have undergone the inherent degradation to which it is subject, even though it was properly stored. For the vast majority of drugs, deterioration only results in a lessened effectiveness of the drug. There have been case reports, however, of drug-induced side effects that were due to the ingestion of outdated tetracyclines,[8,9] and there may be other drugs with which this is a potential problem. Thus, the use of a deteriorated drug product can be dangerous not only from the standpoint of ineffectiveness but also because of the side effects peculiar to the decomposition products of the drug. This same danger should be borne in mind when one is considering the cost savings associated with the purchase of larger volumes of prescription or over-the-counter medications. That is, will the medication be used by the patient before it is destroyed by storage?

While the problem of drug interactions is woven into the entire fabric of drug therapy, and the likelihood of a drug interaction occurring was considered when the drug was initially prescribed, there is no guarantee that using a previously ordered medication will not bring about a drug interaction. The patient may have had other drugs added to and subtracted from the total drug regimen during the interval, and the prescribing physician may well believe that the patient does not have any of the previously prescribed drug on hand. Thus, when the patient restarts therapy with a previously prescribed drug without first checking with either the physician or pharmacist, there is the possibility of adverse reactions occurring that had been guarded against when the physician was aware of all the drugs the patient was using. Although some patients may be reluctant to admit to taking "old" drugs, most would probably be willing to admit that they had been using a prescription drug that had been legitimately obtained.

In summary, self-medication by persons suffering from self-limited minor medical problems is useful and safe within certain constraints. The patient must be willing to admit that the symptoms being treated are not likely to be cured but are simply being relieved. The patient should also recognize when the self-medication attempt has failed and accept the fact that proper medical care should then be sought. The use of safe, effective over-the-counter drug products for the treatment of certain conditions is probably essential to prevent an overload and collapse of the medical care delivery system. The challenge is that patients must be properly informed and educated relative to the medications which they use in their own self-treatment programs.[16]

SELF-ADMINISTRATION OF DRUGS

Early in this chapter, the term self-medication was also used to discuss the accuracy with which patients take the medications that have been prescribed for them by physicians. The term most currently favored for such discussions is *self-administration*,[20] and the phrase used to measure the ability of the patient to adhere to prescribed regimens is *compliance*. The remainder of this chapter is devoted to the problem of patient compliance with both drug and other treatment regimens as prescribed by physicians, a problem that has given birth to an ever-enlarging literature.[1, 10] It is not the purpose of this chapter to review the literature of the entire field, as this has been done by Gillum and Barsky[10] and by Hussar.[13]

Once the patient yields to the unrelenting discomforts of his or her condition and decides to seek medical care, several influences begin to operate to determine the level of compliance that the patient will practice. The patient's first choice is simply not even to begin to comply with the physician's recommendations. This usually means not getting the prescription filled for one of several reasons. Patients sometimes go to physicians expecting to obtain a prescription for a specific pharmaceutical product, and, when this is not prescribed, the patient simply chooses not to take what he regards as an inferior drug product. Such occurrences are probably most often encountered when the patient is seeking a tranquilizer or antiobesity drug. In such circumstances, the attitude of the physician toward the patient's request can exert a negative influence on the likelihood of the drug therapy being followed. Indeed, the attitude of the physician toward the patient himself and his likelihood of following the physician's instructions can exert a negative influence on the patient's compliance with the prescribed regimen.[29]

The cost of the prescription can exert a powerful influence on whether or not the drug is ever obtained initially. This may be a special problem when the patient expects some third-party payment mechanism to handle the cost of the drug. Many patients expect Medicare or group hospitalization insurance programs to cover outpatient prescriptions, which at this time are not generally paid for except through patient reimbursement procedures. Occasionally, the structure of an individual state's Medicaid program is such that some drug products are not covered by the program. In these instances, the patient is often both mentally and financially unprepared to pay for the medication and may simply refuse to fill the prescription due to the lack of financial resources. On other occasions, the patient may expect to pay for the medication but is not prepared to pay the amount of money that is required. This may result in either total refusal to fill the prescription or in the patient's obtaining only a portion of the medication.

Sometimes, because the patient finds it difficult to locate a drug product, he gives up on the physician's selection of therapy. The problem of locating the drug can occur with recently marketed products which have not yet been fully distributed to area pharmacies or in cases where the drug is rarely prescribed and the pharmacy stock has been exhausted and not replenished due to oversight on the part of the pharmacist. Sometimes chemical ingredients in prescriptions which must be compounded may be difficult to obtain, and the patient may not be able to have the prescription filled. An example of difficulty in locating a drug product occurred in 1975 with the marketing of ibuprofen (Motrin®) by the Upjohn Company. Sales predictions and production runs for the product, prior to marketing, turned out to have greatly underestimated the actual market for the drug, and many patients experienced difficulty in locating it when given prescriptions or as refills were needed. This problem persisted for several months, and some patients simply gave up on the medication since they were not able to secure adequate supplies of the drug.

Even when the prescription is filled, problems can exist with the patient being able to take the medication. The Poison Prevention Packaging Act requires the use of child-resistant containers for both over-the-counter and prescription medications.[30] Many elderly patients have found the operation of these containers difficult and quite frustrating and some have smashed them out of frustration at not being able to open the vials. Medications were no doubt destroyed or containers discarded as a result of efforts simply to get to the medication. A call for extensive modification in the requirements of the packaging of dispensed prescription drugs has been made in an effort to simplify the use of the containers by the elderly.

A similar problem with getting to the medication can be seen in the use of certain specialized administration devices for delivery of the medication. Some medications are packaged in aerosol containers designed for oral inhalation, and their use can be confusing although not difficult with practice. Another medication requires the crushing of a capsule in a device equipped with a fanlike unit which the patient activates by inhaling vigorously, thereby pulling the powdered medications into the lungs. Each of these devices often requires demonstration for the patient in order to insure that they are properly used. There are some persons who refuse or resist the use of rectal suppositories or ointments, and an occasional patient misuses a vaginal preparation. Even a seemingly simple act such as putting an ophthalmic ointment into the eye can be frustrating to the patient who is not really sure just how it is to be done. Of course, any drug that must be injected in order to be effective presents the problem of either the patient being able and willing to inject the drug himself or finding a companion who can make the injections on a regular basis. Solving either problem can be difficult and frustrating, particularly for physically impaired or isolated older persons.

The vast majority of medications are, however, for oral solids and liquids and do not present problems of administration. They can present a problem if the patient is unable to understand the instructions for taking the drug. The patient must be able to read the label of the prescription container. While this may not seem to be a problem at first, the pharmacy may use a typewriter that uses either very small type or a script style the patient with poor vision has trouble reading. Some patients may have such poor vision that standard typewriter print is simply unreadable, no matter what the actual style. Many pharmacists also place the label of the prescription container inside the bottle when tablets and capsules are dispensed. If the color of the container is either amber or green, the increased opaqueness of the bottle may be sufficient to make it difficult for the patient to read a label that would otherwise be no problem.

Even if these factors present no problem to the patient, there are some persons who have a basic difficulty in reading and understanding what they have read. Educationally disadvantaged persons, persons of foreign backgrounds, or those who do not speak English as their primary language may all have trouble understanding the label, even though it is clearly printed. Indeed, one study has demonstrated that, even though the pharmacy label was quite clearly and neatly prepared, two-thirds of the patients could not correctly interpret the directions to the prescribing physician.[21]

The pharmacist may also fail to make the labeling explicit enough for some patients who might use oral drops in the eyes or ears, who might ingest suppositories, who would insert suppositories without first removing the protective foil covering, and other seemingly impossible methods of drug product administration. A relatively frequent misadministration occurs when patients swallow tablets designed for sublingual (dissolved under the tongue) or buccal (dissolved in the pouch of the cheek) use. Similarly, some tablets should be chewed before being swallowed, because failing to do so may diminish their effectiveness.

Each patient is also likely to provide his own interpretation of the meaning of the frequency with which medication is to be taken during the day. Each of the most common label instructions for taking medication is subject to individual variation. Does once a day mean once every twenty-four hours, or can it be interpreted as one a day at any time of the day? Several common terms show some of the possible interpretations:

Twice a day—every twelve hours, with breakfast and dinner, with breakfast and lunch, or at 9 AM and at 9 PM
Three times a day—every eight hours, with meals, after meals, before meals, or at unevenly spaced times during the day
Four times a day—every six hours, before or after meals and at bedtime, or on the hospital schedule of 9 AM, 1 PM, 5 PM, and 9 PM
Every four hours—four or six times a day, or maybe even three or five times a day

From the above illustrations, it can be seen that even seemingly clear, well-defined medication administration instructions are subject to interpretation by the patient.

Some may wonder if the adherence to a given frequency of dosing is important, and the only answer that can be given is an emphatic *yes*. Most drugs have well-established patterns of absorption and effect, and these characteristics of the drug were considered when the dosage recommendations were originally formulated by the manufacturer. With many drugs, the maintenance of a consistent blood level is essential to maintain either an adequate level of effectiveness of the drug or to prevent periodic peak levels that place the patient in toxic states. Some authors have suggested that periodic monitoring of blood levels of certain drugs is not only useful in assessing the patient's response to the drug therapy but also to identify and, to some extent, quantify the problem of noncompliance in individual patients.[25] The nature and type of packaging in which the prescription is dispensed can also exert an influence on the ease and reliability with which the patient can be expected to follow the prescribed regimen.[19]

Some of the more important determinants of the accuracy with which patients comply with treatment regimens seem to be the understanding the patient possesses of the disease state, the reason for treatment, the nature of the treatment, and the likely outcome of the condition when the treatment program is faithfully followed.[3, 11, 17, 23] The patient may prematurely discontinue the medication when the discomforting symptoms have disappeared, even though the condition being treated is not completely cured. This is particularly a problem in the treatment of streptococcal infections, since the symptoms usually abate quite early in the treatment program, and the patient does not follow the entire ten-day course of therapy.[19, 23] This problem can often be handled by proper education of the patient to the need to take the full quantity of the medication.

Some patients do not utilize prescribed tranquilizers and sleeping medications due to an inappropriate fear of becoming habituated to the medication. The same is often true of analgesics and other classes of medication noted for their abuse potential. This reluctance to utilize the medication can easily mean that the patient does not get the benefit from the drug that should be obtained, and the problem that was originally being treated only becomes worse. Some patients, however, may expect more from the medication than it can realistically be expected to provide. These patients may discontinue the medication as a result of being dissatisfied with the results that they perceive as accruing from the use of the medication. This problem also must be handled through adequate patient education. The patient must know what benefits can and cannot be expected as result of the drug therapy. If possible, certain signs should be explained to the patient that can be detected to determine either success or failure of the drug. For example, the arthritic patient who can remove a wedding band over a previously swollen joint has been given a positive sign that the medication being taken to relieve inflammation is working.

Every medication has the potential to produce side effects of either a minor or major nature in any patient. Some drugs rarely cause any side effects that the patient could detect, while others regularly produce troublesome adverse effects, such as headaches, dizziness, or diarrhea. The development of an unexpected side effect or the severity of an expected adverse reaction may be grounds, to the patient, to discontinue the medication.[5] A patient should be warned if the medication has the potential to discolor the urine or stool, to cause unusual sedation, to provoke gastrointestinal disturbances, or to cause visual disturbances. The patient should feel better, rather than worse, as a result of his treatment. To do otherwise constitutes grounds for stopping the treatment program and probably undermines the patient's confidence in his physician.

The treatment of chronic medical conditions presents a special problem in maintaining patient compliance with treatment programs. Diseases such as congestive heart failure, essential hypertension, diabetes mellitus, rheumatoid arthritis, and certain pulmonary conditions are treatable and controllable but not curable. This means that the patient must understand that his disease can be slowed down or even halted in its normal pathological course but can never be totally cured. Usually, the treatment of these chronic conditions requires that the patient actively participate in the treatment program in order for successful treatment to take place. Patient education is essential in such circumstances. Often, the prescribing physician must make some bold, effective first step to gain the patient's confidence in the ability of the physician and available treatment regimens to lessen the discomforts of his disease. Such actions as the relief of pain, the return to function of body parts, or cosmetic improvement in dermatological conditions can be important to the patient and act to cement the physician-patient relationship needed in the treatment of chronic conditions. The severity in the change of the patient's life-style that may be required as a part of the treatment can serve as an indicator of the likelihood of noncompliance being a problem.[4] Despite all of the influences on compliance discussed above, the reason most often stated by patients is simply forgetting to take the medication.[24]

No discussion of drug therapy for persons on long-term medications or on multiple medications is complete without some consideration of the cost of drug therapy. It has already been mentioned that the cost of the medication can have a great deal of influence on whether or not the medication prescribed is ever procured by the patient. Most papers on drug costs emphasize the price differentials that exist between brand name and generic drug products. This subject has many facets and has been treated so widely in many other publications, so no attempt is made to cover all the various points of discussion at this time. It is generally true that prescriptions written for drug products by their generic name are less expensive, although the savings vary greatly between pharmacies and depend on the drug prescribed.

There are other ways of saving money on drug costs that are independent of the generic-trade name controversy. One method is for the patient's physician to select the cheapest agent from a pharmacological group of drugs that are essentially therapeutically equivalent. For example, among the various digitalis glycoside products that could be prescribed, digoxin is usually the cheapest and most widely available agent. Thus, prescriptions for digoxin are dispensed for less money than the equivalent dosage amount of some other digitalis products that could be prescribed. Other drug classes and the agent that is generally the cheapest of the group include the thiazide diuretics (hydrochlorothiazide), tranquilizers (chlorpromazine), antihistamines (chlorpheniramine or diphenhydramine), broad-spectrum antibiotics (tetracycline HCl), thyroid hormones (powdered thyroid), anticholinergics (belladonna and phenobarbital), and laxatives (milk of magnesia). It must be emphasized that the selection of the specific drug to be taken by the patient depends first on the drug that will be most likely to successfully treat the condition from which the patient suffers. Only when, in the opinion of the physician, an alternative agent can be used with success are such drug product selections appropriate. Price alone should never dictate the selection of drug products.

The decision to prescribe a drug by its generic name or to select the cheapest member from a class of therapeutic agents belongs, almost exclusively, to the physician. While the patient may express a desire for generic prescriptions, the patient cannot act on his own to procure generic drug products. There are some steps, however, which the patient can take to reduce drug costs that do not require the explicit action of the physician. One important method is the purchase of chronic medications in quantities. Most pharmacists charge less per tablet or capsule for full, original containers than for smaller amounts that must be repackaged. Only in unusual circumstances is the approval of the prescribing physician required to permit the patient to purchase long-term medications in full bottles of one hundred rather than in containers of sixty, as originally prescribed. Bulk purchasing can be overdone, however. The patient should not purchase more medication than can be taken during the normal shelf life of the medication. It would also be prudent to ask the physician who prescribed the medication if any changes in drug therapy are anticipated before purchases of very large quantities of medication to insure against purchasing a drug that is going to be discontinued in the very near future. Pharmacists are forbidden, by law, from accepting dispensed medication for return to stock and reissue to another patient on a subsequent prescription. Thus, the patient who purchases a large quantity of medication may be left with drugs he cannot use or return when the drug is taken out of his therapeutic regimen.

In addition to prudent actions in the purchase of the drug products, selection of the pharmacy for use by the patient can control certain aspects of drug costs indirectly. By using a pharmacy near his or her residence, travel costs may be reduced, and this can be especially so if the pharmacy offers a delivery service and makes no special charge for the delivery of medications. Many insurance and other third-party payment programs require proof of purchase of prescriptions and related items in order for payment to be made. Some persons may find that using a pharmacy that keeps such records as a part of its normal routine can actually save them both time and money through the ready availability of these records without the patient having to maintain the records on his own. Finally, some pharmacies may not participate in a given program of third-party payment in which the patient is enrolled. Every opportunity should be taken to locate a pharmacy that participates in the insurance programs available to the patient. There are many ways, in addition to the procurement of generic drugs, that are available to help control drug costs.

SUMMARY

This chapter has reviewed the total spectrum of the use of medications by the elderly from the standpoint of what the patient can and cannot do to influence his own drug therapy. Beginning with the idea that certain medical problems can be handled with drugs obtainable without a prescription, through the difficulties of following the prescribed treatment regimen, and into the costs of drug therapy, it has been the author's intent to illustrate the obvious and not-so-obvious problems of using drugs properly. Elderly patients frequently take large numbers of drugs for long periods of time, and the proper utilization of these medications can be crucial in the maintenance of good health and well-being.

REFERENCES

1. Ball, W. L.: Symposia on compliance. *Can Med Assoc J, 111*:268, 273, 274, 282, 1974.
2. Compton, W. A.: Self-medication with over-the-counter drugs. *Med Mktg Media, 8*:28-33, 1973.
3. Curtis, E. B.: Medication errors made by patients. *Nurs Outlook, 9*:290-291, 1961.
4. Davis, M. S.: Predicting non-compliant behavior. *J Health Soc Behav, 8*:265-274, 1967.
5. Dixon, W. M., Stradling, P., and Wotten, I. D. P.: Out-patient P.A.S. Therapy. *Lancet, 2*:871-872, 1957.
6. Donegan, T. J.: Role of the Federal Trade Commission in regulating over-the-counter drug advertising. *J Drug Issues, 4*:232-237, 1974.
7. Duckham, J. M. and Lee, H. A.: Vicks vapour rub intoxication. *Postgrad Med J, 51*:115-116, 1975.
8. Frimpter, G. W., Lumpaneli, A. E., and Eisenmenger, W. J.: Reversible "Fanconi-Syndrome" caused by degraded tetracycline. *JAMA, 184*:111-119, 1963.
9. Fulop, M. and Drapkin, A.: Potassium-depletion syndrome secondary to nephropathy apparently caused by "outdated" tetracycline. *N Engl J Med, 272*:986-989, 1965.
10. Gillum, R. F. and Barsky, A. J.: Diagnosis and management of patient compliance. *JAMA, 228*:1563-1567, 1974.
11. Griener, G. E.: The pharmacist's role in patient discharge planning. *Am J Hosp Pharm, 29*:72-76, 1972.
12. Hodes, B.: Non-prescription drugs: An overview. *Int J Health Serv, 4*:125-139, 1974.
13. Hussar, D. A.: Patient non-compliance. *J Am Pharm Assoc, NS15*: 183-199, 1975.
14. Johnson, N.: Junkie television (drug advertising). *J Drug Issues, 4*:227-231, 1974.
15. Kanter, D. L.: Research on the effects of over-the-counter drug advertising. *J Drug Issues, 4*:223-226, 1974.
16. Lasagna, L. C.: The future of clinical pharmacology. *Milit Med, 134*: 477-492, 1969.

17. Latiolais, C. J. and Berry, C. C.: Misuse of prescription medications by out-patients. *Drug Intell Clin Pharm,* 3:270-277, 1969.
18. Lesshafft, C. T.: An exploration of the pharmacist's role in outpatient clinics. *J Am Pharm Assoc, NS10:*205-208, 1970.
19. Linkewich, J. A., Catalano, R. B., and Flack, H. L.: The effect of packaging and instruction on out-patient compliance with medication regimens. *Drug Intell Clin Pharm,* 8:10-15, 1974.
20. Lucarotti, R. L., Prisco, H. M., Hofner, P. E., and Shoup, L. K.: Pharmacist coordinated self-administration program on an obstetrical service. *Am J Hosp Pharm,* 30:1147-1152, 1973.
21. Mazzullo, J. M., Lasagna, L., and Griner, P. F.: Variations in interpretation of prescription instructions: The need for improved prescribing habits. *JAMA,* 227:929-931, 1974.
22. McHale, M. K. and Canada, A. T.: The use of a pharmacist in obtaining medication histories. *Drug Intell Clin Pharm,* 3:115-119, 1969.
23. Moller, D. N., Wallin, D. G., and Dreyfus, E. G.: Studies in the home treatment of streptococcal disease. *N Engl J Med,* 252:1116-1118, 1965.
24. Moulding, T.: Preliminary study of the pill calendar as a method of improving the self-administration of drugs. *Am Rev Resp Dis,* 84:284-287, 1961.
25. Sheiner, L. B., Rosenberg, B., Monathe, V. V., and Peck, C.: Differences in serum digoxin concentrations between in-patients and out-patients: An effect of compliance. *Clin Pharmacol Ther,* 15:239-252, 1974.
26. Tice, L. F.: Safe and sane use of over-the-counter drugs. *Am J Pharm,* 145:187-188, 1973.
27. Walters, P. G.: F.D.A.'s program to improve consumers' and health professionals' ability to select medically effective drugs. *Hosp Form Mgmt,* 9:17, 1974.
28. Weiss, J. and Catalano, P.: Camphorated oil intoxication during pregnancy. *Pediatrics,* 52:713-716, 1973.
29. Wilson, J. T.: Compliance with instruction in the evaluation of therapeutic efficacy. *Clin Pediatr,* 12:333-340, 1973.
30. Wood, R.: Quest for a really safe closure system. *Mfg Chem Aerosol News,* 44:22-23, 1973.

Chapter 9

CLINICAL AND ADMINISTRATIVE ASPECTS OF DRUG MISUSE IN NURSING HOMES

Doris Lang Thomas, M.S.C.

THE ENTIRE SUBJECT of patient abuse in nursing homes should be, and is, a matter of great public concern. The United States is a nation whose culture has assumed the responsibility of caring for the aged. Medicare and Medicaid funding has climbed from millions to billions of dollars in just one decade, but, by and large, the quality of care and service in nursing homes is a failure in public policy. Unfortunately, public concern about nursing home abuses is cyclical, but the demand for improvements should be insistent and constant.

The most recent display of public hand wringing and political lip service occurred in the recent Moreland Act Commission Investigations in New York State.[2] As a result of these hearings, new laws were passed by the New York State Legislature.[3] To the dismay and disbelief of many in the voluntary sector of the nursing home field, the resulting regulations have punished the innocent and have effectively let the guilty go free. Some of the facts to be considered are as follows: (1) The Senate Subcommittee on Long-Term Care was established in 1960. (2) The United States Special Commission on Aging was appointed in 1961. (3) In addition, a steady proliferation of other governmental agencies and private groups have become involved with the quality of institutional care of the elderly population. All have contributed massive documentation to the already well-known litany of nursing home abuses.

More than fifteen years have passed, and the abuses which all the preceding commissions, committees, and citizen groups, both private and public, were intended to combat are scarcely modified. The special prosecutor in the Moreland Commission investigations has asked for indictments for larceny and fraud but none for poor patient care or abuse. Minimal punishment was meted out to the most flagrant offenders, but unscrupulous operators continue to profiteer. Predictable scandals and another round of hearings will probably resurface in due time because the subcommittee estimates that at least 50 percent of homes are substandard with one or more life-threatening conditions.

Drug abuse and misuse is one of the prime areas of offense in long-term care institutions. Some of the findings of the Subcommittee on Long-Term Care[4] indicate the following:

1. The average nursing home patient receives seven different drugs a day, with many being taken up to four times daily. Although physicians are required by law to review the skilled nursing facility patients' medications every thirty days, physicians frequently reorder medications month after month without ever seeing or examining the patient.
2. Approximately 40 percent of the drugs prescribed are for analgesics, sedatives, and tranquilizers. Of this number, half are for tranquilizers. Given normal clinical need for tranquilizers, this suggests a vast overuse of this class of drugs, which probably indicates that most are being prescribed for the purpose of lessening the work load of employees. The use of tranquilizers as "chemical straightjackets" can render alert and ambulatory residents helpless, undemanding, and confined to bed or wheelchair.
3. Drug distribution systems are ineffective and inefficient. The lack of an adequate professional nursing staff often results in aides or orderlies administering medications. Medication errors, which are defined as the wrong drug, wrong dose, wrong patient, wrong route, missed dose, or wrong time, average 30 percent of all drug administrations in nursing homes. This definition applies only to those who administer the medications; it does not include the physician who may prescribe the wrong drug or the pharmacist who can dispense in error.
4. Inadequate drug control encourages theft for personal use or sale. Medication orders are sometimes not termi-

nated when the patient dies or is discharged or transferred, and when such drugs are permitted to accumulate, they often become the property of employees. Furthermore, medications are often charted as if they had been administered when, in fact, they were diverted by unscrupulous employees.
5. Because most nursing homes do not employ the services of an inhouse pharmacist, kickbacks are widespread. It is estimated that 35 percent of the cost of each prescription is paid back to the nursing home operator. The report further indicated that 65 percent of all pharmacists dealing with nursing homes had actual experiences with this method of extortion.
6. The medical and pharmacy community are not attentive enough to the special effects of medication on a geriatric population. The high incidence of adverse drug reactions and drug interactions occurs because of a reduction in metabolic activity, altered central nervous system response, and reduced renal function.

Since governmental agencies have not really seriously addressed themselves to enforcing federal guidelines and specifications for compliance, individual institutions, therefore, establish their own philosophy and then tailor policy and procedure to fit it. If, on the administrative level, a humanistic approach to the care of the elderly is to be the goal, then the residents must be granted a degree of individual dignity and independence, despite institutionalization. This discussion is based on the author's experience within an institution (Isabella Geriatric Center, New York City) with a philosophical base of deep commitment to the needs of this segregated population. The recognition of the necessity to include a pharmaceutical service as a contributing factor in the delivery of adequate medical care is an indication of implementing the goal.

PHARMACY PRACTICE WITHIN A GERIATRIC SETTING

The practice of pharmacy within a geriatric setting is a relatively new concept for the pharmacy profession. The opportunities afforded us are unique, because there was, until a few years ago, little documentation and few references to use as guidelines for geriatric pharmacy practice other than the myriad and often conflicting and repetitive governmental regulations. Drawing on a traditional educational system, however, for an awesome amount of theoretical knowledge and some practical proficiency and on various community and hospital sources, pharmacists can be pioneers and innovators in this emerging specialized field. Because gerontology is establishing itself as a new specialty, pharmacy can and must become an active participant with other professions in the delivery of quality care. In addition to providing the mechanics of the distribution of drugs, pharmacists must become involved with the medical, social, and philosophical aspects of geriatric care. The practice of geriatric pharmacy is a health service and, therefore, patient oriented. With this approach, the drug abuse of nursing home patients, whether deliberate or unintentional, can be prevented.

The Isabella Geriatric Center consists of three separate units: (1) a residential facility, (2) an intermediate care facility, and (3) a skilled nursing facility (nursing home). Following are several examples of how the pharmacy department of the Center participates with other disciplines to prevent drug abuse.

Pharmacy is represented on the Admissions and Transfer Committee where basic decisions are made concerning the appropriate placement of new applicants and those who are already in residence. The rendering of pharmacy services is directly related to the required level of care. The pharmacy department is also an active participant of the Pharmacy and Therapeutics Committee. Physicians, nurses, administrators, and pharmacists together develop written procedures and policy for effective drug therapy and related matters.

The pharmacy department reviews the drug regimen of intermediate care facility residents at least every sixty days with the medical clinic nurses and physicians. The department also participates in the thirty-day review of the drug regimen of each patient in the skilled nursing facility. It is required by law that any irregularities be reported to the medical director and the administrator. In addition, the pharmacy department provides the psychiatric staff with a periodic review of psychotropic drugs prescribed for the nursing home population. In accordance with the philosophical beliefs of the institution, the nursing, medical, and pharmacy staffs work together to insure a minimal dosage level of these medications. This permits maximum patient participation in programs and activities instead of overmedicated residents being allowed to vegetate because of a chemical straightjacket.

The pharmacy department is responsible for providing schedules to the other departments to insure the continuity of the thirty-day review of medications and special orders for nursing home patients. Before Medicare and Medicaid review became mandatory, the pharmacy department instituted, along with the medical, nursing, social services, and dietary departments, a modified "rounds" program through which individual cases were reviewed. Pharmacy, along with other departments, alerts the social service department regarding behavioral and social problems of any resident.

Finally, the pharmacy department is a monthly participant in an ongoing nursing inservice training program. Topics are selected on the basis of pertinence to Isabella Geriatric Center's geriatric population. The educational process is reciprocal, in that the pharmacists learn from nursing observations and, therefore, are more aware of drug responses.

The physical location and arrangement of the pharmacy department is also felt to facilitate effective clinical pharmacy administration. The pharmacy department is located on the second floor of the facility. This floor is shared with medical clinics, occupational therapy, physical therapy, the dentist, the X-ray department, podiatry, the beauty parlor and the barber shop, nursing offices, and social service. The medication needs of the residential and intermediate care facility residents are served within the pharmacy compound.

The waiting room leads into two consultation rooms, one for the residential facility dwellers and the other for intermediate care facility residents. An individual consultation room offers a comfortable, dignified atmosphere in which the pharmacist can communicate with residents concerning the nature of their illnesses and help them to understand the use of their prescribed medications.

Since pharmaceutical services at Isabella Geriatric Center are based on the unique needs of the Center's three distinct levels of care, these services will be discussed separately for each population. Each of these discussions focuses on the interrelated and interdependent procedures of drug distribution and monitoring.

PHARMACY SERVICE TO RESIDENTIAL FACILITY DWELLERS

Isabella House, the geriatric center's residential facility, is designed for the independent living of relatively well older persons able to maintain themselves adequately in their own apartments. The population of the house is approximately 250, and the average age is eighty-four. In addition to the established rental, there is a service plan package cost which, among other services, includes a medical plan and prescription medications. The delivery of pharmacy services here closely parallels community pharmacy dispensing. In addition, a major component of medication management at the Isabella Geriatric Center is the maintenance of a patient profile card, which includes information on the patient's age, diagnosis, allergies, personal physician, and history of medication use. When a house resident presents a new prescription or a refill request to the pharmacist, the patient's profile card is automatically checked first. However, as in community pharmacies, it is not possible to maintain full supervision of drug use by these residents because they are not required to use the Center's medical staff. They may engage an outside physician and/or select another pharmacy. In addition, nonprescription medications are beyond staff control. Despite these exceptions, the profile card system proves adequate enough to monitor to a large extent duplicate and discontinued drugs, last refill, number of refills, and so on.

When the patient presents his doctor's prescription, the medication request is noted on a daily work sheet indicating patient name, apartment number, prescription name, strength of medication, and pickup time. An appointment slip is then issued to the resident as a written reminder of (1) prescription order date, (2) number of prescriptions ordered, and (3) date and time for pickup (this is usually same-day service). When the prescriptions are completed by the pharmacist, a charge slip is affixed to the bagged order. Upon presentation of the appointment slip, the charge slip is matched. The medication is then discussed with the house resident, and a signature of the resident is affixed to the charge slip. The slip serves a two-fold purpose in that it provides the pharmacy with a daily accounting system and proof of pickup. At the end of each day, a pharmacist reviews patient charts in the medical office for any change in the drug regimen of those residents who utilize the house physician and adjusts the patient profile cards to reflect those changes. This is done primarily to prevent the inadvertent refill of a prescription which has been discontinued for some reason by the physician.

PHARMACY SERVICE TO INTERMEDIATE CARE FACILITY RESIDENTS

The next area of pharmacy service to be considered is that delivered to the intermediate care facility population. This facility houses 207 residents whose average age is eighty-five. An intermediate care facility resident may be described as a person who requires institutional care to secure basic services necessary to maintain various degrees of independence. Historically and currently, the nursing department administers medications to this group. The customary procedures in many facilities may include (1) residents queuing up before entering the dining room to be given prepared doses which must be ingested immediately, or (2) the nurse going from table to table in the dining room during mealtimes with the prepared medications cups, or (3) residents remaining roombound until the nurse is able to service them. There are exceptions to these traditional methods of distribution. The New York State Code allows self-administration of medication with the written permission of the resident's attending physician. Approximately ten years ago, after the Isabella Geriatric Center's pharmacy department was installed and organized, a decision was made to inaugurate a program of self-administration of medication. It was, and still is, an acknowledgement of our commitment to the preservation of individual dignity and independence. The pharmacy department, together with the medical, nursing, and social service departments, developed procedures for such a program. To a large extent, the successful achievement of this goal is dependent upon an exacting monitor system, clear and concise labeling of medications, an empathetic pharmacy staff, and constant resident education through counseling. A recently published report of the Study Commission on Pharmacy concluded:

> Clearly, pharmacists must have ready knowledge about drugs but they must also have ready knowledge about people, about relationships and communication with them. The Study Commission reiterates the point that pharmacy is a knowledge system in which chemical substances and people called patients meet and interact. Needed and optimally effective drug therapy results only when both drugs and those who consume them are fully understood.[1]

The pharmacy department receives a social history of each new admission. This preintroduction serves as a guideline for future observations. Members of the Center's staff endeavor to establish a personal relationship with every resident. An awareness of his personality, attitude toward illness, attitude toward taking medications, and degree of attention and concern required help to establish a healthy patient-pharmacist association. Because of constant contact with the intermediate care population, there are many opportunities to observe behavior and behavioral changes. This information is then shared at various interdepartmental committee meetings. An example of how such information resulted in a decision of the Admissions and Transfer Committee is that of Mr. S.:

> Mr. S. is a seventy-eight-year-old widower who had worked in the garment industry from his youth until retirement. He "loved the ladies," enjoyed "dressing smart," and reminisced about winning gold trophies in dance contests. Despite his present physical disabilities, he still managed to maintain a flirtatious mood and an attractive wardrobe. He needed and used the pharmacy service frequently, and our relationship was mutually warm and friendly. Approximately two years after admission, Mr. S. began to exhibit social and attitudinal changes. His clothes gradually became rumpled and sometimes soiled. He "forgot" to shave. He was pleasant when spoken to, but seemed withdrawn and vague. He was discussed at resident review meetings where the dietary and nursing departments concurred with the observations of the pharmacy department. The social service department continued to counsel him after several psychiatric sessions, but unfortunately, he deteriorated

further. He was unable to comply with his medication regimen, needed assistance in all activities of daily living, and became increasingly confused. Mr. S. was finally transferred to the skilled nursing facility.

The remainder of this section is devoted to a description of the system of dispensing and monitoring medications for this resident population.

Those intermediate care residents who qualify for self-administration (and at present only 4 out of 207 do not) are provided with medication boxes complete with their names, the pharmacy location and business hours, and instructions for prescription filling. This box is a convenient method of storage of all the patient's medications and can be carried with the patient if a temporary transfer to the nursing home is required. The residents bring their prescriptions from our medical clinic to the pharmacy. Pharmacy hours are scheduled to coincide with clinic hours when the doctors are available for consultation when required. The waiting room is shared by both residential and intermediate care facility populations, but each resident is serviced in a private consultation room, which provides a good opportunity for instruction of the patient in the appropriate use of his medications. Their prescriptions are filled while they wait.

A daily review of the patient profile card is again utilized as a control measure. This card includes an additional column to check off the retrieval of the prescription container, since pharmacy policy dictates that no prescription is refilled without the return of the empty container. (Although this system protects against inadvertent patient errors, it does not prevent conscious attempts to hoard unused drugs.) Moreover, because most of these residents are permitted to administer their own medications, several drug categories (primarily maintenance medications) require special surveillance, including (1) cardiac drugs, (2) hypertensives, (3) diuretics, (4) diabetic drugs, (5) steroids, and (6) psychotropics. Maintenance medication amounts are dispensed in cycles for seven-, fourteen-, and twenty-eight-day supplies, depending on the patient's ability to comply. New residents start with a seven-day supply which may, when appropriate, be increased. Most patients are comfortable with a seven-day cycle, feeling that small amounts are easier to count and handle. A special monitor card indicates the date on which the patient is scheduled to return for a refill of his medication. These cards provide us with an early warning system of patient noncompliance. Copies are forwarded to the physicians, the clinic nurse supervisor, and the department of social service.

Although a successful system of communication with the receiver of medication—whether it is patient or nurse—is important for the residential population, it is absolutely essential for residents of the intermediate care facility. This is achieved primarily by means of a legible, instructive, and informative label. Labels should be typed in capital letters using two-tone ribbons for special emphasis. The signa (drug name and directions for use) of a prescription can be defined in terms of what, when, how, and why. The *what* is the drug identity, strength, and quantity. The *when* is the descriptive period of the day or week, rather than a specific time. Pharmacy department experience indicates that if specific times, such as 9 AM, are stated on the label, especially for maintenance medications, the patient becomes too anxious. The time is interpreted literally, and there is a deep concern about punctuality. Many of our patients need reassurance that a fifteen- or thirty-minute deviation from the stated time is not calamitous. Thus a signa of "Once a day" becomes "In the morning"; "Twice a day" becomes "In the morning and in the evening"; and so forth. The *how* denotes special instructions. A tetracycline prescription written as "Four times a day" becomes "Take one capsule four times a day one hour before meals and at bedtime with water only." The *why* states the intention of use. Hence, a prescription written for indomethacin to be taken three times a day translates to "Take one capsule three times a day with meals for arthritic pain." Pharmacy policy dictates that no prescription may be dispensed with a signa indicating "Use as directed" or "Use as needed," so physicians who give such orders must be contacted for adequate instructions.

The amount of dispensed medication plus the signa results in instant information to the pharmacist on patient compliance. However, some residents lack normal manual dexterity and have impaired vision, which may account for possible mathematical shortages due to spillage rather than noncompliance. In addition, a continuous effort is made to select medications and containers with varied colors and shapes for easier identification, and a red heart emblem is affixed to every cardiac medication.

Finally, many residents enjoy visiting the pharmacy and socializing with the staff. In addition, many residents are reassured by their ability to use medication properly, and those with marginal memory are proud of their ability to remain independent. A good illustration of this phenomenon is the case of Mrs. P.:

> Mrs. P. was admitted to the skilled nursing facility as a Medicare patient. After her recovery from surgery, she was transferred to the intermediate care facility. Although the resident was able to cope with activities of daily living, the diagnosis indicated mild organic brain syndrome. Her medication regimen included two monitored medications and one laxative, and we programmed her on a seven-day cycle. Fortunately, Mrs. P. was mildly compulsive, and appeared in the pharmacy every Friday morning at 10 AM for refills of the monitored drugs.

PHARMACY SERVICE TO SKILLED NURSING HOME RESIDENTS

The third area of pharmaceutical service is that provided to the skilled nursing facility population. The nursing home is for aged persons in need of regular and continuing nursing supervision and medical care. It is primarily for residents who can no longer manage in the intermediate facility. It is also a certified skilled nursing facility under the Medicare and Medicaid programs. The population consists of 315 patients whose average age is eighty-six years.

The present system for drug distribution and monitoring is a result of gradual changes and refinements. When the pharmacy service was established, drug distribution continued with the traditional bulk-drug floor-stock system. Since old methods are usually well entrenched, the involvement of the nursing department and the administration was crucial in effecting new concepts and procedures. After many meetings, a modified unit-dose system was instituted and, with it, a system of accountability.

The existing nursing units were equipped with individual medication boxes, and floor by floor the conversion was accomplished. At that time, the skilled nursing facility totaled 120 residents with forty beds per floor. A few years later, another opportunity to evaluate the system occurred when the institution decided to expand. A new building was being planned to include an enlarged skilled nursing population to total 315 beds. The pharmacy department again decided to investigate alternative methods of distribution and monitoring. Together with the nursing department and with administrative approval, a pilot project with a cart service was instituted. The project was a joint venture between the nursing and pharmacy departments, which met and discussed their particular needs and requirements. Finally, nursing and pharmacy procedures were revised so that the cart became a portable service system. The back of the cart is divided into two sections, one of which, for purposes of security, is double locked to accommodate controlled substances, while the other contains all internal floor stock. The carts are serviced weekly by schedule, and medications are dispensed by this method to seven nursing home floors with forty-five patients per floor. The institution of the cart concept enabled the elimination of expensive nursing units, which saved the administration thousands of dollars.

The areas of responsibility for drug dispensing in this manner are clearly defined. The nursing department orders floor stock and supplies biweekly. Because Isabella Geriatric Center is approved for a New York State Schedule 3 License, these scheduled drugs are also dispensed as floor stock. The nursing department initiates new prescription orders by submitting to the pharmacy department a duplicate requisition sheet on which has been transcribed the information from the physicians' order sheets. These order sheets must also accompany the requisition. The physicians' order sheet is then checked by the pharmacy department for medication and dosage, and the patient profile is examined for allergies, diagnosis, duplication, and drug interactions. The orders are then copied by the pharmacist from the original physicians' order sheet onto the patient profile card along with an indication of the length of time that a medication may be administered based on the legislated thirty-day review. Quantities of drugs for short-term therapy are determined by either the physician's order or the automatic stop order. This is a policy set by the Pharmacy and Therapeutics Committee establishing the maximum length of time that a medication may be continued (in the absence of a physician's specification) before it is automatically stopped. Again, the container retrieval feature of the patient profile card is utilized to remove discontinued drugs and prevent the accumulation of containers when patients die or are transferred or discharged. Now the prescriptions are ready for processing. Replenishing the cart is a pharmacy function.

CONCLUSION

The pharmacist, because of specialized knowledge, must become an active, working partner in the delivery of quality health care. Where else can the standards of professionalism be better manifested than in a long-term institution? Because of the stationary population and a dedicated, multidisciplined staff, the ideal practice of pharmacy can become a reality.

REFERENCES

1. Millis, J.: *Pharmacists for the Future.* Report of the Study Commission on Pharmacy. New York, National Foundation for Medical Education, 1975.
2. Moreland Act Commission: *Past Lapses, Future Prospects: A Summary Report of the Moreland Act Commission on Nursing Homes and Residential Facilities.* Albany, New York, Moreland Act Commission, 1976.
3. New York State Legislature: *Long-Term Care Regulations,* Section 6, 1976.
4. U.S. Senate Subcommittee on Long-Term Care of the Special Committee on Aging: *Nursing Home Care in the United States: Failure in Public Policy.* Supporting Paper No. 2: *Drugs in Nursing Homes: Misuse, High Costs, and Kickbacks.* Washington, D.C., U.S. Govt Print Office, 1975.

Section III

CLINICAL AND COMMUNITY RESPONSE TO ELDERLY DRUG USE

Chapter 10

THE PHYSICIAN'S ROLE IN THE ADMINISTRATION OF PSYCHOTROPIC DRUGS TO THE ELDERLY PATIENT

WILLIAM F. WIELAND, M.D.

THE AVAILABILITY OF drugs that influence behavior has revolutionized the practices of mental health professionals. Many people can not only be more effectively treated than previously, but this treatment can usually be administered without the need for hospitalization or at least without prolonged hospitalization. It has taken longer, however, to learn how to use these drugs with equal safety and efficacy in the elderly and to teach nonpsychiatric physicians to recognize these disorders in the elderly so that they can either prescribe appropriate treatment or make appropriate referrals.[2-8]

Furthermore, the drugs that influence behavior are still too often prescribed injudiciously, especially the sedatives and minor tranquilizers, and they are often used equally injudiciously by untutored or uncontrolled patients. Since elderly people often seek drugs to cure their various ills and since physicians often have a compulsion to provide such drugs, the elderly frequently become unwitting victims of drug misuse or abuse.[2, 5-7] While there has been a huge amount of national concern over drug abuse among youth, there has been insufficient attention paid to patient-initiated or iatrogenic drug abuse among the elderly.[3, 4]

This chapter explores some of the types of behavior in the elderly that may be responsive to drugs, the types of drugs that are most apt to be effective, and some practices to be avoided.

CHARACTERISTICS OF THE ELDERLY

Aging per se is not a disease: It is not preventable and does not require drug treatment. As with any other stage of life, there are normal stresses, expectations, capabilities, and vulnerabilities peculiar to this stage. It is a striking observation that age-specific factors are well understood and usually well tolerated in infants, children, adolescents, young adults, and middle-aged adults, but they are frequently misunderstood and poorly tolerated in the elderly. This is at least one of the reasons why such factors are so poorly managed in many elderly people.

Some of the common age-specific psychological factors in the later stage of life are fear of death, loneliness, uselessness, and changes in body image and self-concept. There are also typical physical changes, such as decreased muscular power, slower reaction time, poorer visual and hearing acuity, reduced sexual drive or performance, and changes in sleep patterns. These changes, as well as many others, are part of the normal process of aging to which each individual may respond in a relatively healthy and mature manner or with varying degrees of maladjustment or psychopathology.

In addition to the normal stresses of normal aging, there are various disorders affecting behavior that primarily occur during this stage of life, including senile dementia, cerebral arteriosclerosis, paranoid reactions, depressive reactions, and confused or delirious states. All of these disorders may be mild, moderate, or severe and may be acute, intermittent, or chronic in nature.

Finally, elderly people experience changes in their normal economic and social support structure. There is an inevitable decimation in the ranks of their friends and relatives; their children may be widely dispersed geographically and, at any rate, are preoccupied with their own family activities; their previous occupations are either terminated or markedly reduced. These factors, too, place an additional burden or need for adjustments on people at a time of life when such adjustments are often difficult to make.

Based on the above brief description of changes and stresses, it is not difficult to understand why elderly people suffer from various emotional and behavioral disorders. The difficulty lies in the ability to assess and treat these disorders as safely and effectively as possible.

MAJOR DRUGS USED TO INFLUENCE BEHAVIOR

There are a large number of drugs that influence behavior, and this influence may be in a positive or negative direction.

All of these drugs are two-edged swords and, therefore, must be carefully selected and monitored in each case. Most of the drugs that influence behavior can be classified as *sedatives* (barbiturate and nonbarbiturate), *stimulants* (amphetamines, methylphenidate, and caffeine), *major tranquilizers* (phenothiazines, haloperidol, and thiothixene), *minor tranquilizers* (meprobamate and benzodiazepines), *antidepressants* (tricyclics and MAO inhibitors), *lithium carbonate,* and *analgesics* (narcotic and non-narcotic). *Antihistamines* may also have behavioral effects although they are not usually prescribed for that purpose, except for their use in the elderly as mild sedatives (Table 9-I).

Each of the seven classes (or eight if antihistamines are included) of drugs are effective for relatively specific symptom relief. Generally speaking, a particular symptom or disorder does not respond to a drug in the wrong class, and the person receiving the wrong type of drug is apt to remain as ill as before or show further deterioration from side effects. It is true that each of these drugs has some general systemic or nervous system effects which may provide additional benefit or harm over and above its effect on specific symptoms. It should be emphasized that the appropriate selection of a drug requires considerable knowledge of the pharmacology of each one, as well as a careful assessment of the target symptoms requiring treatment.

This chapter is not designed to be a short course in pharmacology, but it should be underscored that four of the seven classes of behavior-influencing drugs are particularly susceptible to abuse. These four are sedatives, stimulants, minor tranquilizers, and analgesics. All of these drugs rapidly alter one's state of consciousness; all are capable of producing tolerance, thereby requiring larger doses to produce the desired effect; all but the stimulants produce physical dependence when used at higher doses on a daily basis. Therefore, it is particularly important to prescribe these four classes of drugs judiciously, preferably for short periods of time, and with adequate instructions to the patient and his family of the risks of abuse. Drug addiction is not confined to youth, and it can just as easily occur with well-intended prescription drugs as it does with illicit drugs.

Another precaution is in order before discussing the treatment of specific disorders. There has been a dangerous trend toward

TABLE 9-I

COMMONLY PRESCRIBED DRUGS WHICH INFLUENCE
BEHAVIOR IN THE ELDERLY*

Type of Drug	Useful In	Adverse Effects
1. *Antidepressants* Imipramine (Tofranil) Desipramine (Norpramin, Pertofrane) Doxepin (Sinequan) Amitriptyline (Elavil) Nortriptyline (Aventyl)	Depression and depression with anxiety	Delirium Psychosis Hypotension Cardiac arrhythmia Agitation Mania
2. *Major Tranquilizers* Chloropromazine (Thorazine) Trifluperazine (Stelazine) Thioridazine (Mellaril) Fluphenazine (Prolixin®) Haloperidol (Haldol®) Thiothixene (Navane®)	Paranoia Agitation	Drowsiness Delirium Hypotension Parkinson-like syndromes
3. *Minor Tranquilizers* Chlordiazepoxide (Librium) Diazepam (Valium) Meprobamate (Equanil®, Miltown®)	Anxiety reaction Transient situational reaction	Delirium Equilibrium disturbance Habituation **Addiction** Withdrawal
4. *Hypnotics* Chloral hydrate (Noctec®) Barbiturates Ethchlorvynol (Placidyl) Methyprylon (Noludar®) Flurazepam (Dalmane®) Methaqualone (Quaalude®, Sopor(TM))	Anxiety reaction Transient situational reaction Other sleep disturbances	Delirium Habituation Addiction Withdrawal Suicidal tool
5. *Stimulants* Methylphenidate (Ritalin®) Amphetamines		Hyperstimulation Habituation Addiction
6. *Analgesics* Aspirin Acetaminophen (Tylenol®) Pentazocine (Talwin) Opiates (natural and synthetic)	Pain	Stimulation Sedation Addiction Withdrawal
7. Lithium carbonate	Mania	Lithium toxicity
8. Antihistamines	Sleep disturbance	Drowsiness Confusion

* Adapted from E. Pfeiffer, Use of Drugs Which Influence Behavior in the Elderly: Promises, Pitfalls, and Perspectives. In R. H. Davis and W. K. Smith (Eds.), *Drugs and the Elderly*. Ethel Percy Andrus Gerontology Center, U of S Cal, Los Angeles, 1973.

polypharmacy or the "shotgun" approach in treating people with psychiatric or behavior disorders. It is not uncommon for these people to receive three or more drugs on a regular and prolonged basis. As a rule of thumb, one or two appropriately selected drugs at an appropriate dosage accomplishes more than multiple drugs and does so at less risk to the patient and at a lower cost. If one or two drugs are not doing the job, one should first consider changing the drug or the dose before adding other drugs to the regimen.

Finally, before prescribing any drugs, it is essential to obtain a drug history to determine what drugs have been used before, whether they were helpful or harmful or neither; what drugs are currently in use and whether they are helpful or not; what over-the-counter drugs are used; and how reliable the patient has been in taking prescribed medication. A rational and effective treatment plan cannot be devised without this information.

COMMON PSYCHIATRIC DISORDERS IN THE ELDERLY

All psychiatric disorders may occur in elderly people. These may represent a recurrence of previous disorders or may be a continuation or further deterioration of a chronic disorder. It is, however, not uncommon for a disorder to occur for the first time during one's latter years, and several disorders are particularly prevalent. These are described briefly, including general recommendations for appropriate drug treatment.

Depressive Reactions

The most common psychiatric syndrome in the general population as well as in the elderly is depression. The elderly are particularly vulnerable to depression because of the numerous losses they experience and because there is less future time available to compensate for the losses. The symptoms of depression include physical complaints, sleep disturbances, appetite disturbances, lack of energy or drive, sadness, and pessimism. All of these symptoms may be mild to severe and may either be isolated or associated with other physical disease or senile changes, etc. They may also be associated with increased alcohol or drug consumption. The appropriate treatment may only require supportive counseling, including family members or friends; it may involve the use of antidepressants, particularly tricyclics, where the symptoms are more severe or of long duration; it may involve hospitalization. These decisions rest on a careful assessment of the whole patient and a determination of the availability of various environmental supports. It is usually best to avoid the other classes of behavior-altering drugs, although mild sedation or mild tranquilization may be helpful for *short* periods of time. One should always inquire about suicidal ideation in depression, but it is especially important in the elderly, since they account for about one-third of all suicides in the United States.

Paranoid Reactions

Paranoid reactions are generally less serious than similar reactions in younger people, but they are often extremely annoying to families and friends. They tend to occur when the elderly person is also suffering from mild dementia, hearing loss, or a major change in environment. The paranoid ideas usually involve neighbors or friends, but they may be more cosmic in proportions. The treatment in most cases includes stabilizing the environment and helping the family or friends understand and cope with the paranoid ideas. Frequently, the use of relatively *small* doses of a major tranquilizer produces excellent results. It is important in most cases *not* to prescribe sedatives or minor tranquilizers, since these drugs further reduce cortical functioning and thereby tend to increase the paranoia and the sense of isolation.

Confused or Delerious Reactions

Confused or delerious reactions are most apt to occur with cerebral arteriosclerosis, but they may occur with any organic brain deficit. They are often precipitated by illness, surgery, or drugs. Treatment is nonspecific and should include support, reassurance, reduced stimulation, and sedation. If there is an underlying physical disorder, this should be corrected whenever possible.

Agitation

Agitation is a common symptom, but it is usually associated with other reactions such as depression, paranoia, or anxiety.

When it is associated with depression or paranoia, appropriate treatment of the primary condition usually reduces the agitation. Sometimes a second drug, such as a minor or major tranquilizer, may also be needed for short periods. When agitation is primarily due to anxiety, supportive counseling and intermittent use of minor tranquilizers may be helpful.

Sleep Disturbance

Sleep disturbance is a common symptom in all psychiatric disorders. It must be remembered, however, that normal sleep patterns in the elderly tend to show less stage 4 (deep) sleep and more frequent awakenings. There is also a greater tendency to require some sleep during daytime hours. Since these are normal changes with aging, it is usually only necessary to help the patient adjust to the changes and accept them. Seldom, if ever, should sedative drugs be prescribed to influence what is essentially a normal process.

Pain

Many elderly people suffer from joint pain or pain related to other somatic disorders. Since most of these sources of pain are long-term or chronic in nature, it is essential to prescribe analgesics judiciously, starting with the mildest drugs, such as aspirin, and using more potent drugs only on an as-needed basis or for brief periods. Pain is very troublesome to the patient, his family, and the physician, but much benefit can be gained by all parties when it is assessed carefully, when the limits of treatment are carefully explained, and when the use of potent, addicting analgesics are avoided except when truly needed. Terminal illness associated with severe pain need not be treated as cautiously.

Organic Brain Syndromes

Organic brain syndromes include arteriosclerotic brain disease, which usually affects the specific brain areas where blood supply is restricted; senile brain disease, a diffuse process of cell death throughout the brain; and presenile dementia, which is the same as senile dementia but occurs earilier in life and is extremely rare. Drug treatment in organic brain disease is used only to reduce specific target symptoms such as depression, paranoia, agitiation, or severe sleep disturbance. It should be done with the full knowledge that good results are less predictable and that side effects are often more troublesome.

Hypochondriasis

Although hypochondriasis can occur at any age, it is particularly common in the elderly. It may be seen in relatively pure forms where there is no significant underlying psychiatric or somatic disorder, or it may occur as a symptom of other disorders. In the latter case, most of the effort should be devoted to treatment of the underlying disorder. In the pure form, however, it is necessary to hear the patient out, provide supportive counseling, and improve the living situation if possible. Hypochondriasis is a plea for help and should be responded to accordingly. It does *not* usually improve by using powerful drugs, and these should be avoided. In fact, many hypochondriacs are already taking excessive medication, and the appropriate treatment in these cases is to stop this practice.

ASSESSMENT

There are a number of ways to assess a person's psychological, emotional, and behavioral status. A simple way to categorize this assessment is as follows:

1. Cognitive or intellectual functions, including intelligence and any deterioration thereof, presence or absence of thought disorders (hallucinations, delusions, blocking), associations (tight or loose), memory (recent and remote), and signs of aphasia, agnosia, etc.
2. Affective or emotional functions such as depression, anxiety, irritability, fear, hostility, agitation, and euphoria
3. Attitudes toward oneself, toward relatives and friends, toward the examiner, about the past, and about the future
4. Behaviors such as seclusiveness, hoarding, avoiding activities, eating habits, sleeping habits, irritating other people, etc.

A careful evaluation of the four functions provides important clues for proper diagnosis, prognosis, and appropriate treatment.

It also provides a baseline against which to evaluate improvement or further deterioration.

There are many times that a physician is so preoccupied with the treatment of physical disorders in elderly patients that the behavioral or psychiatric disorders are neglected. This neglect deprives the patient of optimal treatment, sometimes to the detriment of the physical ailment as well, and often prevents the attainment of optimal relationships between the patient and other significant persons who must share his burdens. The additional time it takes to learn how to assess psychiatric disorders in the elderly and to prescribe drugs appropriately greatly enhances the quality of life for all concerned parties.

CONCLUSION

Powerful new drugs have greatly enhanced the ability to treat psychiatric disorders in all age-groups. But, being two-edged swords, they have also created new problems which we must continue to address. Unfortunately, there have been too few programs established to educate physicians, mental health professionals, and the public in both the benefits and the problems created by the availability of such drugs.

Since the majority of elderly people live in the community, major efforts should be devoted to the proper education of physicians, nurses, and pharmacists. These are the people most likely to be in a position to assess behavioral disorders and to be the purveyors of licit drugs. Therefore, they are the keystone both for providing optimal treatment and for preventing misuse or abuse.

The elderly residing in hospitals or nursing homes are much more dependent upon the staff of these institutions, who may be more concerned about making their jobs easier than about the welfare of their patients. This frequently results in administering excessive or inappropriate drugs.[1] Such practices need to be addressed by a combined approach of education and of better mechanisms for monitoring and peer review.

There is no simple solution to the numerous behavioral problems of the aged any more than there is for any other stage of life. The tools are better than ever before but are still far from perfect and in some cases are not effective at all. Nevertheless, much can be done by people who have sufficient knowledge and the commitment to do an effective job. There is no doubt that a great deal of needless suffering would thus be alleviated.

REFERENCES

1. Barton, R. and Hurst, L.: Unnecessary use of tranquilizers in elderly patients. *Br J Psychiatry, 112*:989-990, 1966.
2. Bourne, P. G.: Drug abuse in the aging. *Perspect Aging, 2*:18-20, 1973.
3. Davis, R. H. and Smith, W. K. (Eds.): *Drugs and the Elderly.* Los Angeles, Ethel Percy Andrus Gerontology Center, U of S Cal, 1973.
4. Fann, W. E. and Maddox, G. L. (Eds.): *Drug Issues in Geropsychiatry.* Baltimore, Williams & Wilkins, 1974.
5. Pascarelli, E.: Alcoholism and drug addiction in the elderly. *Geriatric Focus, 11*:1, 4-5, 1972.
6. Pascarelli, E. F. and Fischer, W.: Drug dependence in the elderly. *Int J Aging Hum Dev, 5*:347-356, 1974.
7. Pfeiffer, E.: Use of drugs which influence behavior in the elderly: Promises, pitfalls, and perspectives. In Davis, R. H. and Smith, W. K. (Eds.): *Drugs and the Elderly.* Los Angeles, Ethel Percy Andrus Gerontology Center, U of S Cal, 1973.
8. Wynne, R. D. and Heller, F.: Drug overuse among the elderly: A growing problem. *Perspect Aging, 2*:15-18, 1973.

Chapter 11

NURSING RESPONSIBILITIES IN THE ADMINISTRATION OF DRUGS TO OLDER PATIENTS

JAMES A. THORSON, ED.D.
JUDY R. J. THORSON, R.N., M.ED.

THERE ARE FEW areas where the uses of the nurse's skill and judgment are more important than in the administration of medications. The nurse is the person responsible for seeing that the therapeutic program called for by the physician is carried out. Frequently, the nurse is also the person on the health care team who has the greatest amount of contact with the patient and hence the greatest knowledge of his likes and dislikes, idiosyncrasies, and behavior.

The older patient, especially the nursing home patient, sometimes is an angry and frustrating person to deal with. Studies have shown that nurses generally prefer almost any other type of nursing service than with geriatric patients.[10] However, there are few areas of greater need and greater satisfaction for the nurse who is dedicated to the alleviation of human suffering than working in geriatrics. Deep attachments and friendships are often developed; many older persons are reservoirs of wisdom and are genuinely interesting people. Talking with and listening to the reminiscences of older people was one of the really enjoyable parts of the authors' geriatric nursing experience.

Although only about 4 or 5 percent of the population over the age of sixty-five is institutionalized at any one time, it is a fact that most nursing care delivered to older adults is in an institutional setting.[3] This chapter deals with drug administration in both the institutional and the community setting. The great emphasis in health care service delivery now and in the future is, properly, in the development of alternatives to the unnecessary institutionalization of the elderly. Since the registered nurse often is in the position of being an administrator rather than a bedside nurse, this chapter is addressed to paraprofessionals as well as to professionals in the nursing field.

It should be remembered by all members of the health care team that chronic conditions make up by far the greatest number of medical problems of older persons. At the turn of the century, pneumonia and tuberculosis were the great killers of the elderly. Other contagious diseases were frequent killers of older patients. Only about 4 percent of the population survived to age sixty-five. In the final quarter of this century, with over 10 percent of the population reaching later adulthood, the conquest of contagious disease is apparent. The leading causes of death in older adulthood are cardiovascular ailments (50%), cerebrovascular problems (15%), and cancer (15%). This means not only that a great proportion of the populace is living into old age but also that a greater percentage will ultimately suffer from one or more serious chronic conditions.

Thus, the health care practitioner, who obviously is in the business of getting people well, may be frustrated in that there are no quick cures for many chronic conditions, and patient progress is slow. In addition, a great amount of physical and psychological suffering is associated with such chronic health problems as heart disease, arthritis, stroke, and cancer. It may be discouraging to realize that the best that modern medicine has to offer may be to temporarily ease the pain caused by an incurable condition. The nurse must also remember a fact that American society all too frequently denies: All patients must ultimately die.

Further, the nurse should be aware of a number of social messages that some elderly persons attach to the taking of medications. Especially if he is institutionalized, the patient who is receiving medication is likely to develop a "sick role." That is, he may play the part, or what he imagines to be the part, of a person who is sick, rather than the part of a well, independent person who is temporarily hospitalized. The institution itself contributes to the development of sick-role behavior.[5] If the patient's perception of a hospital or nursing home is that of a place where people go to die, then a program of rehabilitation for that patient is vastly complicated. Institutions (and nurses) have certain behaviors that reinforce the patient's adoption of the role of a sick, or dying, person. In the extreme example, Glaser and Strauss[11] discuss the problem of the person who is socially dead—the person who is a living organism but who is treated as an object rather than as a person by the institution's health care personnel.

The physician and nurse must be aware of the social message of medications. A tranquilizer, for example, is a pill that is taken by someone who is sick—someone who is anxious or depressed or agitated. A glass of wine, on the other hand, may have exactly the same effect as the tranquilizer but conveys the message of wellness and perhaps of sociability or even celebration.

Aging persons are individuals and should not be lumped into a single category because of chronological age. Drugs, obviously, communicate different messages to different individuals. Some older people do not like to take drugs at all; having to rely on chemical intervention into one's bodily processes is an admission of vulnerability and a loss of autonomy and independence. These persons may prefer to deny a symptom rather than to seek medical attention. Other persons, while not outright hypochondriacs, like to take drugs and enjoy the attention they get from doctors and nurses. Overdosage is sometimes caused by the self-administration of drugs by the individual who feels that "if some is good, more is better."

Keeping the above psychological factors in mind, the nurse should have several goals in the treatment and medication of the geriatric patient:

1. To promote the wellness and independence of the patient
2. To prevent institutionalization of the patient in the community or to help rehabilitate the institutionalized patient and return him to the community
3. To be sure that the physician's program of care is carried out. Specifically, it is important
    a. That drugs are accurately dispensed;
    b. That the proper dosage is administered;

c. That the drugs are actually taken; and
d. That the drugs are not in conflict with any other substances taken by the patient
4. To ease the patient's pain and anxiety
5. To allow the dying patient to die with dignity

DETERMINING PATIENTS' DRUG HABITS

It is vital, especially with the older patient, that previous or current drug habits be determined. The authors recall one elderly patient, newly admitted to a skilled nursing home, who developed acute discomfort because the nursing staff was not aware of his serious laxative dependency. He had taken a large dose of milk of magnesia every day for many years and was in real pain, not to mention emotional anxiety, when this was withdrawn upon his admission to the institution.

Drug abuse, most often with legal substances, is sometimes a problem with the elderly patient. The older abuser of dangerous illegal drugs has been seen infrequently up to the present, probably because the abuse of hard narcotics has been a phenomenon associated with youth in our culture and the fact that few drug addicts live into older adulthood. Capel and his associaates[7] point to the future problems that will develop as the current generation of abusers of hard drugs ages. The fact remains, though, that many older persons have developed a dependency on legal substances such as laxatives, alcohol, or prescription drugs such as tranquilizers. Wynne and Heller[13] report that "nearly one-fifth of the patients entering the geriatric service of a general hospital displayed disorders directly attributable to effects of prescribed drugs."

Persons who have taken drugs for many years and then have them withdrawn upon entering a health care institution may frequently suffer a reaction. Equally serious is the patient in the community who is responsible for self-administration of multiple prescriptions. For this reason, it is very important that the nursing assessment of the patient, whether or not he is institutionalized, include a history of the over-the-counter and prescription drugs that the patient has been taking.

The nurse should be aware that the patient may have prescriptions from several physicians and that these drugs may not all be compatible or that the patient may be taking two or even three times as much of a drug as is necessary. In addition, the prescription may have been meant for a limited time and the patient, not understanding, has continued to refill and take a medication that is not needed. The assessment of the patient's drug habits should also include patient preferences for administration; some persons prefer to take medications with fruit juice or in applesauce rather than with water.

OBSERVING POSSIBLE SIDE EFFECTS

Illness and institutionalization are major stresses in an older person's life. The side effects of medications can add to and compound the older patient's problems in coping with stress. Not only may patients have a reaction to drugs they have taken, but they may react to the institution or environment itself. The generation that is now aged grew up at a time when the poorhouse or county farm was the last stop for the hopeless; they may associate admission to a nursing home with these past concepts and withdraw into an isolated existence. Symptoms of disorientation can often be explained by the new environment. A person who upon awakening in the middle of the night is not able to find the bathroom might appear to be hopelessly confused. In actuality, he may have been patterned over fifty years to turn right when getting out of bed to go to the bathroom and have a hard time adjusting to a situation where he must turn to the left. Symptoms similar to drug reactions may also be caused by the environment that the patient has just left. Eisdorfer[9] reports on the misdiagnosis of a series of elderly patients who were admitted for psychiatric hospitalization when their real problem was dehydration.

The nurse should of course be observant of drug reactions or side effects caused by allergies, conflicting prescriptions, and overdose. The nurse is frequently the first person to notice such interactions, and it is the nurse's responsibility to report any untoward symptoms to the physician.

Tolerance of certain drugs is lower in the elderly. According to Citrenbaum,[8] the liver has an important effect in detoxifying drugs, and decline in liver function may allow too high a dosage of medication to enter the body. Also, a lessened amount of liver bile leads to a tendency for a decrease tolerance of fat and a decreased absorption of vitamins A, D, E, and K, the fat-soluble vitamins. Foods may have a reaction with certain drugs. Blumberg and Drummond[2] report that "monoamine oxidase inhibiting drugs react with foods that contain amines such as cheese or yogurt to produce an acute hypertensive crisis."

Many elderly persons suffer from too many drugs rather than too few. Many persons arrive at the hospital or nursing home with a bag full of medications, and a drug baseline needs to be established for them. Further, overdose is a serious problem because of decline in liver function, a decline in physical activity, and loss of weight. The standard dose for an average well individual may be lethal for an older person. Again, the nurse must take responsibility to insure that the physician is aware of the possibility of overdose in the prescription of medications for older patients.

It is unfortunate but true that some older patients, especially in nursing homes, are the victims of oversedation because of the nurse's recommendation. Behavior problems are all too frequently solved by overtranquilizing the patient. In some of the early research on victims of Parkinson's disease using L-dopa, it was observed that nursing problems were created when the patients' conditions improved. Previously inactive and withdrawn patients became much more aware of their environment and reacted by complaining about poor food and nursing service. The temptation with patients who are causing problems with the nursing staff is to sedate them, and physicians are frequently willing to follow the nurse's recommendation for prescriptions of tranquilizing drugs. Ironically, Anderson[1] has noted that the overuse of sedatives may lead to other nursing problems: confusion, sleeplessness, incontinence, and accidents. Also, the long-term effect of such sedation is very serious. Butler and Lewis[6] state, "Unfortunately drugs reinforce some of the slowing observed in old people, aggravate a sense of aging and depression, and can contribute to or directly cause acute and chronic brain syndromes."

To prevent unnecessary reactions and to reduce the amount

of drugs given, the nurse should use nursing measures before resorting to medications. Causes of restlessness, such as noise, light, temperature of the room, uncomfortable bed clothes, fear or loneliness, and hunger or thirst, respond much better to proper nursing intervention than to sedation. The patient should be allowed to use his own home remedy, such as hot water or honey and lemon juice, if it will help him to get to sleep. The nurse can also help the patient to sleep at night by keeping him from dozing off in the daytime. Institutionalized patients frequently do not get the physical activity they need to induce a sense of tiredness. Hodkinson[12] maintains that "recourse to sleeping tablets should be considered an admission of failure on the part of the nurse to interest, occupy, and feed the elderly person properly."

DRUG ADMINISTRATION

The unit-dose system has been a great aid to the nurse who may be responsible for administering drugs to fifty to sixty patients, many of whom are receiving more than one medication. Obviously, the nurse should take care that the right drug is given to the right patient. Further, the nurse should notify the physician if a particular prescription is unreasonable; physicians are frequently under severe time constraints and mistakes do happen. A patient's life may depend on catching such a mistake, and no one expects the physician to be infallible, popular television portrayals notwithstanding.

The nurse should be aware of a number of factors that influence the administration of drugs. One such factor is that many older patients do not like to take drugs. Medications may upset the stomach, and gastric juices frequently are diminished; at least half of a glass of water should be given with oral medications. Also, the social message the patient gets when given a pill may not be a pleasant one. Persons who have lived through fifty or even sixty years of responsible adulthood are sometimes confronted by a nurse young enough to be their grandchild proffering their pills, with the implication that the older person is not capable of taking care of his own drug administration. Such role reversal is sometimes interpreted as an indignity, and a few older patients react by behaving according to the implied expectation and becoming obstreperous, hoarding pills, or refusing to take their medications.

The nurse should be sure that the patient does in fact take the drug but should also administer it in such a way as to maintain the patient's dignity and self-respect. Older persons are not drug-taking machines and have decreased reaction time and difficulty in swallowing a number of pills. They should not be rushed and should not be talked down to or treated as a child. A patient's questions should be answered as completely as possible; he should not be told, "Because it's good for you," when he has asked why he is being given a certain medication.

Ten to twenty percent of medications are not given orally. The nurse should be aware that the older patient has lost much subcutaneous fat, that the skin is looser, and that connective tissue is resistant to injections, causing difficult penetration and pain. Anderson[1] recommends that it is safest to give injections in the buttock rather than in the thigh or deltoid. The nurse should check frequently for pain and inflammation.

Elderly patients may require pain medication on a regular basis for chronic conditions. The nurse, acting as the patient's advocate, should establish a basis of trust with the patient so that he knows he can rely on the nurse to administer pain medication faithfully and regularly. Patients who do not receive pain medication when it is scheduled or when they have requested it often react against the nurse whom they hold responsible for their unnecessary pain. Blumberg and Drummond[2] maintain that pain medications should ". . . be given regularly and in amounts large enough to relieve pain. It is unwise to have pain medication on a prn ("take as needed") pattern because this pattern places too much responsibility on the patient to ask for medication. Rather, pain medication should be given regularly around the clock. In this manner, often smaller doses of the narcotic are needed."

The nurse has the responsibility of interpreting the patient's pain to the physician and not withholding prn doses when the patient needs them. Patients may develop a fear, when having to request prn medication, that they may have to wait for it or, even worse, that they may be forgotten. Brown[4] says that establishing a climate of trust eases the situation for both patient and nurse: "If the pain-ridden individual is assured that he will not be permitted to suffer from pain, he loses his anxiety. Having faith that the nursing-medical team will prevent the recurrence of pain, he is much more able to live through long periods of severe pathology before a peaceful death occurs." The nurse should be aware that proper positioning of the patient in the bed, as well as physical activity, can prevent much pain.

PATIENT SELF-ADMINISTRATION OF DRUGS

Most geriatric patients continue to live in the community outside of institutions. Therefore, most medications taken by older persons are self-administered. The nurse has an important educational and counseling function to perform with the person who is responsible for the self-administration of drugs—or who will be responsible upon discharge from an institutional setting.

Of primary importance is that the patient knows why he is taking a particular medication, when he should take it, and under what conditions it should be taken. The authors recall one elderly woman who took tranquilizers regularly for a four-year period. Her physician had prescribed them for her when her husband had died, and she did not realize that they were to be taken only during the period of her immediate grief.

The nurse can work with the pharmacist and physician to be sure that all prescription drugs are labeled clearly in large type with the name of the drug, what it is used for, possible side effects, the proper dosage, and the expiration date. Correct usage of drugs depends on the patient's knowledge of what he is taking and why. Also, Butler and Lewis[6] state that, "There is another safety factor in adequate labeling. When the doctor cannot be reached or the pharmacist's records are in error, good labeling makes it possible to check on medications if allergic or other untoward reactions occur. The old person or another family member, often a child, may unwittingly take an overdose of a drug or take the wrong drug."

Patients should be warned against mixing two different kinds of drugs in the same bottle. It is the nurse's responsibility to determine the patient's ability to administer his own medications and to report any problems to the doctor. Where the patient needs assistance, the nurse can help to devise a plan for assistance from family members or home health aides. Frequently, patients who are sometimes forgetful can successfully administer their own medications if they have been provided with written instructions and reminders.

One reminder may be a chart posted near the medications in the patient's home that allows the patient to check off when he has taken his pills. Other aids include a printed clock with color-coded instructions or an egg carton with different medications for the day assigned to separate compartments. Many birth-control pills now come in containers that indicate whether or not the daily pill has been taken; such containers could be used with imagination to help solve some of the drug-taking problems of the elderly. What works for one patient may not work for another, and the nurse should take the time to be sure that the patient learns the proper routine and schedule for his medications. In addition, a family member should understand the older person's drug regimen.

GERIATRIC NURSING CARE

Many problems older persons have with drugs can be avoided with good nursing care and patient knowledge. An example of a situation where the patient's understanding of his condition and its treatment could have avoided trouble is that of a hypertensive patient on a low-salt diet who frequently took Alka-Seltzer® (which is very high in sodium) for headaches. A good educational program can prevent such problems. It is the nurse's responsibility not only to teach the patient the correct routine for his own drug-taking behavior, but also to warn him of the dangers and uselessness of many over-the-counter preparations.

Good nursing care involves the maintenance of a trusting relationship with the patient. Physicians frequently do not have the time to adequately explain conditions and treatments. Such explanations from the nurse can relieve much patient anxiety.

Sitting at the bedside, maintaining eye contact and perhaps touch with the patient provides valuable reassurance for patients who often feel that the medical staff is not particularly interested in their problems.

Unfortunately, we are too eager to turn to drugs to handle human relations problems. Many physicians give newly bereaved persons sedation unnecessarily. According to Butler and Lewis,[6] "Suppression of a symptom—be it depression or anxiety—may be undesirable. For instance, in a depression viewed as a maladaptive expression of grief, the release of suppressed grief will have a more enduring value than drug-suppressed depression. No drug can substitute for a lost loved one, as therapeutic counseling and the forging of new relationships can."

The nurse should be aware of the geriatric patient as a human being in a social setting. Just as good physical care can prevent bedsores, human contact and good listening behavior can ease anxiety and depression.

REFERENCES

1. Anderson, H.: *Newton's Geriatric Nursing*. St. Louis, Mosby, 1971.
2. Blumberg, J. E. and Drummond, E. E.: *Nursing Care of the Long-Term Patient*, 2nd ed. New York, Springer Pub, 1971.
3. Brickner, P. W. (Ed.): *Care of the Nursing-Home Patient*. New York, Macmillan, 1971.
4. Brown, M. I.: Nursing of the aging and aged. In Chinn, A. (Ed.): *Working with Older People*. Vol. 4. Public Health Service, Publ. No. 1459, Washington, D.C., U.S. Govt Print Office, 1971.
5. Burnside, I. M. (Ed.): *Psycho-Social Nursing Care of the Aged*. New York, McGraw-Hill, 1973.
6. Butler, R. N. and Lewis, M. I.: *Aging and Mental Health: Positive Psychosocial Approaches*. St. Louis, Mosby, 1973.
7. Capel, W. C., Goldsmith, B. M., Waddell, K. J., and Stewart, G. T.: The aging narcotic addict: An increasing problem for the next decades. *J Gerontol, 27*:102-106, 1972.
8. Citrenbaum, M.: *Drugs and the Elderly from the Point of View of a Nurse*. Paper presented to The Drugs and the Elderly Conference, Georgia State University, Atlanta, February 17-19, 1975.
9. Eisdorfer, C.: The impact of scientific advances of independent living. In Thorson, J. (Ed.): *Action Now for Older Americans: Toward Independent Living*. Athens, Georgia, U of Georgia Pr, 1972.

10. Gillis, M.: Attitudes of nursing personnel toward the aged. *Nurs Res,* 22:517-520, 1973.
11. Glaser, B. G. and Strauss, A. L.: *Time for Dying.* Chicago, Aldine, 1968.
12. Hodkinson, M.: *Nursing the Elderly.* Long Island City, New York, Pergamon, 1966.
13. Wynne, R. D. and Heller, F.: Drug overuse among the elderly: A growing problem. *Perspect Aging,* 2:15-18, 1973.

Chapter 12

STRATEGIES AND TECHNIQUES FOR DRUG EDUCATION AMONG THE ELDERLY

RONALD J. GAETANO, B.S., R.PH.
BETSY TODD EPSTEIN, R.N., B.S.N.

THE PATIENT IS the least knowledgeable member of the health team, and yet the patient is the person who must coordinate his or her own health care. It is the patient who decides whether or not to seek care; the patient who initiates contact with the health care system; the patient who provides much of the input with which the health team makes decisions; and the patient who chooses whether or not to follow the prescribed medical regimen. Unfortunately, the patient is not usually given enough information to safely and effectively handle his or her responsibilities as a member of the health team. The difficulties that many elderly individuals encounter in managing a medication regimen illustrate the dangers of this unbalanced system. One way to approach the problem is through a consumer drug education program.

DEFINITION OF THE PROBLEM

The fastest-growing segment of the population in the United States is made up of people over the age of sixty-five. Of approximately 22 million people in this age-group, over 95 percent are living in the community and monitoring their own health care at any one time.[22] Their self-medication includes the administration of prescribed drugs (carrying out a physician's order without direct medical or nursing supervision) and the selection and use of nonprescription drugs. In our experience, a good deal of this self-medication is carried out in an uninformed manner, resulting in unsafe or ineffective administration of the medicine. In a 1962 study of medication errors made by elderly, chronically ill ambulatory patients, 59 percent of the study population was found to be making one or more errors in self-medication; 26 percent made potentially serious errors.[20]

The Elderly as a High-Risk Population

Medication misuse is a negative health behavior that exists among adults of all ages, but the older person is more likely to experience problems resulting from inappropriate drug use. Although aging is not a disease, the aging process invites chronic conditions and diseases that require chemotherapy. People over sixty-five make up 10 percent of the United States population and consume 25 percent of all prescription drugs.[21] It is probable that the percentage is the same for over-the-counter medication. Brady has stated that the occurrence of adverse drug reactions is directly related to the number and frequency of drug-dose exposures.[1]

Physiological factors contribute to the older adult's increased risk of developing drug side effects and adverse reactions.[12] The rates of absorption, distribution, metabolism, and excretion of drugs tend to decrease with advancing age. The resulting difference in drug activity in the older adult's body yields a different therapeutic response than in the younger adult. Increasing age may predispose to hyper- or hyporeactivity.[13] Either possibility contributes to an increased incidence of adverse drug reactions among the elderly. In addition, the reserve capacities of the organ systems are decreased. It is, therefore, more difficult for the aged body to adapt to stress (such as that resulting from an adverse drug reaction), and a longer time is required for a return to equilibrium.[19]

Complicating physiological problems is the lack of specified geriatric drug doses. Most experimental data on drug metabolism are obtained from adults in their mid-twenties.[4] There is a pediatric dose for most drugs or a formula such as Young's Rule or Clark's Rule for finding the dose.[15] No one has devised similar general guidelines for geriatric prescribing. The normal adult dose of a drug is not always appropriate for elderly patients.

When the drug literature does suggest guidelines for geriatric prescribing, they are often ignored. The literature on Valium recommends an initial geriatric dose of 2 to 2.5 mg once or twice daily to avoid the development of ataxia or oversedation. Yet in our experience, most patients are started on doses of 5 mg one to three times daily.

Problems in geriatric prescribing extend beyond dosage regulation. Some of the drugs most often used with elderly patients exhibit poor risk-to-benefit ratios for their target population. The literature on Indocin® (an antiarthritic drug), for example, notes gastrointestinal, ocular, and central nervous system effects that are particularly dangerous in an elderly patient.[17] When an older adult experiences these side effects, an uninformed physician is likely to attribute them to "old age" rather than to the drug.

Limited dexterity and decreased visual and hearing acuity are present to some degree in most older adults.[19] These impairments can create obstacles in opening medicine containers, reading labels or distinguishing between pills, and hearing instructions. Many of the elderly live alone or with other older people, and there may be no one available to compensate for these kinds of physical deficits.

The inability of the elderly to find health resources is sad. Many senior citizens receive inferior medical care simply because they have lost their doctors through death or retirement. Many are going to overworked physicians with large, long-standing practices, and these patients hesitate to seek new doctors for fear there are none available. The use of emergency rooms for non-emergency problems is one indication of the older adult's precarious ties with the health care system.

In addition, social factors centering around the concept of *loss*—of family and friends, occupation, income, social status, mobility, and health—can make life very stressful for an older person. Characteristically, there are few available alternatives by which he or she can deal with these stresses. The emotional bases contributing to medication misuse are complex, but our own experience and that of other authors indicates that stress can affect the way in which the older person perceives and uses his or her medicine.[6]

Examples of Misuse

Studies done by Schwartz and her associates[20] and Hamm[8] as well as our own experience in working with the elderly point out several common and potentially dangerous self-medication behaviors:

- Lack of knowledge of the name or action of a particular drug
- Lack of knowledge of how a particular drug must be taken to be effective (chewed or swallowed whole, with or without food and so on)
- Lack of knowledge of what constitutes a side effect
- Taking medicines irregularly because of lack of motivation, forgetfulness, expense, or self-determination of need
- "Stretching" medicine to make it last longer than the period for which it was prescribed
- Borrowing and lending medicines
- Saving old medicines and tending to self-treat with these
- Overdosage by the ingestion of duplicate medications prescribed by different physicians
- Mixing different drugs in one container
- Inappropriate use of over-the-counter medicines

General Factors Contributing to Misuse of Drugs

The factors contributing to drug misuse can be discussed by examining the attitudes of the people who most directly affect drug-taking behaviors: the lay public, physicians, and pharmaceutical manufacturers.

In general, lay people's expectations of health care, in particular expectations about the role that medications should play, can contribute to drug misuse. James Isbister,[11] head of the Federal Alcohol, Drug Abuse and Mental Health Administration, has said, "To some extent [drug misuse] is due to a societal attitude that condones, even encourages, the use of medication as a first line of defense against any complaint or symptom, both physical and mental." Among consumers there is a general lack of understanding of how drugs work. The idea that there is a pill to remedy every complaint and that the doctor has failed if he or she is unable to prescribe a *perfect* medication to alleviate the patient's symptoms is unfortunately common. Many people shop around to find a physician who will prescribe what *they* want.

Robert DuPont, director of the National Institute for Drug Abuse, has pointed out that the physician who allows himself or herself to be manipulated by persons seeking drugs can contribute to the problems of drug misuse. Other inappropriate prescribing is done by well-intentioned but not fully informed practitioners.[3] In our experience, a great number of psychotropic drugs are prescribed by physicians unable to cope with the multicomplaint (chronic) patient in any other way. In addition, the medication regimen of the geriatric patient tends to be reevaluated less aggressively (if at all) than that of the younger adult.

Irresponsible advertising on the part of some patent drug manufacturers has contributed to the public's unrealistic expectations of drug therapy and fostered the development of a health mythology. The Food and Drug Administration has had limited success in regulating suggestive advertising,[14] and their recent study of over-the-counter drugs may have some positive effect on limiting exaggerated advertising claims.[10]

Values and Behaviors of Health Professionals

Many health professionals prefer not to work with elderly patients for whom maintenance rather than curative care is the norm. Significant figures from an American Medical Association survey in 1972 illustrate this point. The survey found that there were 18,000 pediatricians to care for the young but fewer than 300 recognized geriatricians.[18]

Some practitioners are blatantly discriminatory in their dealings with older adults and foster stereotypical expectations of aging. Studies of the attitudes of medical students have indicated that they consider older people to be more emotionally disturbed than younger adults, more apathetic, withdrawn, disagreeable, dissatisfied, and disruptive of social and family welfare.[23] "What do you expect at your age?" may be the doctor's response to an elderly person's complaint. Unfortunately, this biased and ignorant attitude contributes to the elderly person's negative self-image and can take away the motivation to comply with his or her medical regimen.

In a dialogue between the doctor and the elderly patient,

the roles of "parent" and "child," respectively, are often assumed. As part of the busy "parent" role, the doctor tends to hurry and spends little time with the older patient. The doctor may not question a patient to learn whether he or she understands a new health condition or medicine, but because of the decrease in visual and hearing acuity experienced by many older persons (and sometimes, in addition, their reluctance to admit any impairment), it is especially important for the doctor to elicit feedback from older patients.

Government agencies and professional groups spend a great deal of time talking to each other about "the problem of drugs and the elderly," but very little is being done to change the behavior of the elderly consumer. As in other human service programs developing today, professionals often make health care decisions while ignoring the target group. The accumulation and exchange of knowledge only among health professionals is selfish and counterproductive.

ONE APPROACH TO THE PROBLEM

Group Health Education

During the past three years, we have worked directly with elderly consumers in separate programs in the northeastern and midwestern United States. It is our belief that, through an educational process, the drug use behavior of the elderly individual can be changed to make it a much more positive factor in his or her life. The process of health education involves the concept of change—in knowledge, attitudes, and finally, behavior.[2] Values and attitudes can be changed when people realize that their present behavior is costing them much in money, health, and well-being.

We suggest that the primary effort should be on reaching the consumer, rather than focusing on significant others or health professionals. An individual cares more about his or her own life than do others and is realistically often in the best position to coordinate his or her own health care. In order to safely and effectively manage health care, the consumer needs more knowledge.

The general objective of a drug education program is to

produce a well-informed patient who has the knowledge that he or she needs in order to develop safe and effective drug-taking behavior. The health professional thus obtains a patient who asks intelligent questions and follows the prescribed chemotherapy with the best possible results. Onek and his associates have observed that increased knowledge leads to increased compliance.[16] Certainly, the greater the health knowledge a patient has, the less is his or her need to improvise in health situations.

While the main emphasis of a drug education program is drug use information, other productive health behaviors can be encouraged. Two ancillary objectives are therefore important to the accomplishment of the main objective: the first is to foster a more positive, prevention-oriented attitude toward health on the part of the consumer; the second objective is to increase the older person's confidence and interest in participating in his or her care plan and in dealing with the health care system.

Designing a Curriculum

An early task of a drug education program is to design a curriculum. Most people over the age of sixty have had little, if any, formal health education. The information (or misinformation) that an older adult has collected through the years has come from friends, relatives, and the communications media—radio, television, newspapers, and magazines. With this fact in mind and after surveying and working with elderly groups, the following pilot curriculum has evolved.

Anatomy and Physiology

Most older adults know little about how the human body functions. A review of basic facts is necessary before beginning any practical discussion of drug use.

Pharmacology

Consumers in general are not aware of the effects that drugs have on the body. Even the most basic facts about his or her own medications have often been omitted from the elderly individual's education. Typically, the drug information the patient needs is not given or it is given but not understood, and the patient is reluctant to ask questions.

The elderly should be made aware of the aged body's slower

rate of food and drug metabolism. It is especially important for the consumer to understand what to look for in therapeutic effects, side effects, and idiosyncrasies.

The subject of drug-drug and drug-food interactions, although difficult even for professionals to understand, should at least be addressed with the senior citizen. An example that is easy for most people to relate to is an explanation of how caffeine and nicotine can interact with a decongestant.

When an individual understands how important his or her daily life-style is to the drugs he or she may take, changes in attitude and behavior are more likely to occur.

Drugs and Disease

The study of diseases and conditions often associated with aging and the drugs commonly employed to control them are involved. By relating dysfunctions to normal anatomy and physiology, the positive aspects of drug use—how drugs can promote a return to homeostasis—can be emphasized. This is an especially important point for health professionals to consider when working to foster a positive attitude toward drugs, particularly since many older adults feel that all drugs produce physical dependence.

Monitoring Personal Drug Use Behavior

Information that is important for the consumer to learn about his or her own medicines includes how and when a drug should be taken, where it should be kept, early warning signs of adverse reactions, and the kinds of feedback physicians need from patients. Pharmacy patient profiles and personal drug profiles are described.

Many people in government and some consumer groups ignore the issue of drug quality to focus on the more visible problem of cost. This attitude is usually based on the erroneous assumption that all medicines are of the same quality and that chemical and therapeutic equivalence is assured. Because of these misconceptions, Food and Drug Administration standards and drug-quality-control measures are detailed in the course. We emphasize the need for high-quality, economical medicine.

We suggest that the implementation of more positive drug use behaviors is an effective way to economize. Studies of specific kinds of health education—for example, preoperative teaching[9]—have shown it to be cost-effective by reducing the hospitalized patient's length of stay. Group health education in the community should promote cost savings by promoting and improving consumer understanding and utilization of medication and local health care resources.[5]

Identification of Available Resources

A general discussion of how the health delivery system works and how the older adult can most fully utilize it is also important. However, it is unwise to create anxieties among group members if we are not prepared to meet those needs. As health professionals involved in consumer education, we feel it is our responsibility to identify those elderly participants who have unmet health needs. Through individual follow-up, we try to ensure that these people reenter the health care system. Some of the older adults do not readily fit into any part of that system, but we continue tracking those individuals to try to learn what alternatives might meet their needs.

Special Projects

Field trips to emergency rooms, hospital wards, and drug manufacturing firms are special projects. The chain of events in a typical emergency room is reviewed. The main points emphasized are to refrain from using emergency rooms for the treatment of nonemergency conditions and to understand the system to avoid needless anxiety when emergency room visits are necessary. In a visit to a hospital ward, we discuss how to understand the rules of the ward and how to use the hospital and its staff to the patient's best advantage. These exposures can reduce the anxieties of the older patient and be indirectly helpful to the health professional when the time comes for the elderly to use these resources.

A visit to a drug manufacturing firm is designed to help people reexamine their values about the cost versus the quality of drugs. With some knowledge of the manufacturing process and the need for quality control, the consumer can put the issues of cost and quality into better perspective. The questions that arise as well as the revelations that occur are encouraging.

Practical Considerations in Educating Older Adults

While individual elderly persons can be difficult to reach (the problem of the homebound elderly is beyond the scope of this paper), the elderly as a group are not. Drug education programs can be instituted in established senior citizen groups or in groups gathered specifically for health education.

Our experiences in both programs have resulted in a delineation of drug education programming into two phases. The first phase involves less formal education to senior citizen groups, while the second includes a more structured curriculum.

Senior citizen groups in any region of the country are fairly visible. Initial contact with established groups in any community can often be made through the local or state agency on aging. The groups with which we have had the most contact have been at nutrition sites, senior apartment buildings, libraries, community associations, and churches and synagogues. These groups welcome speakers at their weekly or monthly meetings.

One advantage of instituting health education in an established group is that the professional can create an environment that makes change (in knowledge, attitudes, and behavior) as easy as possible. These students do not have to take the initiative to seek out health education if it is brought to their regular meeting places. In addition, the friendships that group members have made among themselves can make this setting a very nonthreatening one and one in which it is easier for individuals to ask personal health questions. There tends to be more security for group members in this setting; the consumer rather than the professional is in the comfortable position of control.

There are older adults who enjoy an academic environment and therefore actively seek learning opportunities in the community. More formal adult education can be offered to this group of older adults. In New York State, a minicourse was instituted in a local college to ascertain the interest of the elderly in drug education. The first course was to consist of a core group of twelve so some controls could be placed on this group. The response to a flyer sent to a group of senior centers was so overwhelming that thirty-three people were enrolled in the first course. In the more structured setting of a community college or other local academic network in which the students have already indicated their desire to learn something new, more detailed learning objectives can be set, and actual learning is more readily measured.

In beginning drug education, which is a personal, potentially threatening topic to older adults, it is especially important to choose an instructor who can establish a good rapport between himself or herself and the group. If the audience sees the instructor as part of the medical establishment and not as a caring individual, communication is difficult to maintain and little, if any, learning will take place.

The teacher in any health education program for the elderly should have a positive attitude toward older people in general. An instructor who is younger than the elderly students is not successful if he or she has stereotypical misconceptions about old people. The instructor needs to realize that older students bring a wealth of life experience to any learning situation. Older adults have information to share, and a good teacher recognizes their potential contribution to the learning process.

The discussion following a health talk is often the most valuable part of the session, and it is essential to choose an instructor who has a broad knowledge of health and health care to be able to field questions from the group. Most of the elderly have specific health concerns, and they apply new information to their individual situations. Their questions are very practical. A well-informed and sensitive physician, registered nurse, or pharmacist is usually able to answer such questions to the group's satisfaction. Nurses and pharmacists are probably more suitable (and more easily obtainable) than physicians as health educators; they are certainly more cost-effective.

The elderly are not any more homogeneous than younger populations. Age (the "young-old" and "old-old"), education and cultural backgrounds, financial resources, access to health care, and intragroup relationships differ from group to group. An assessment of "where the group is at" is necessary in order to individualize educational objectives.

Decreased visual and auditory acuity should be taken into account.[7] More than with younger groups, the speaker needs to consciously maintain a clear, moderately paced, low-pitched delivery. The use of audiovisual aids has been kept to a minimum in our programs, primarily for flexibility at the various education sites. Large illustrations are used to supplement the teacher's information. Supplementary materials (handouts) should be in large print and understandable language. Since these materials are not always easy to find, we have printed some of our own supplementary notes in large type and distributed these to the groups. This last point illustrates one of our primary concerns in the health education of older adults: the lack of educational resources available to the consumer.

The supposed short attention span that has caused much concern among those working with the elderly has not presented a problem in our work. The attention span of older adults, in our experience with over 5,000 seniors from widely divergent backgrounds, has been as good as that of high school students. The questions that arise are a good indication of whether or not most of the group has understood the material.

The physical environment for learning should be taken into account. In particular, the meeting place should be accessible with a minimum of physical obstacles such as stairs, transportation needs should be taken into account, and the time of day for meetings considered. In some areas, an evening meeting time may be undesirable for safety reasons.

The initiation of group health education in any community changes the perceived roles of many health professionals. Those who resist sharing health information argue that the patient with more knowledge experiences more health-related anxieties or "causes problems" for the rest of the health team. In our experience, these are invalid assumptions. Information about health and medications, presented in a positive and easily understandable way, serves to lower the anxiety levels of most patients. We suggest that the few patients who find such information anxiety-provoking are people who approach most life situations in an inappropriately anxious manner. These people need health intervention of a different kind. In the majority of older adults, however, we have encountered a demanding and exciting desire to learn more about their health concerns.

The fear that a more knowledgeable patient is a more

troublesome one is unfounded. One advantage of a community-based health education program is the fact that it encourages communication between health professionals and the particular consumers that they serve. Many seniors in our groups have returned to us to report very positive interactions with their own doctors, nurses, and pharmacists; similar comments have been received from professionals. The patient who understands the reasons for his or her medical regimen is often more likely to comply with it.

SUMMARY AND RECOMMENDATIONS

We believe that consumer education should be the main emphasis of a drug education program for older adults. In a program designed to prevent the inappropriate use of drugs, professional education is also necessary. Doctors, nurses, and pharmacists need to be made aware of the special problems of medication use among the elderly. More research in the areas of drug-drug and drug-food interactions is needed, and greater efforts should be directed toward developing geriatric doses for drugs. In addition, health professionals need to devise more efficient ways of disseminating drug information in a quick and comprehensive manner.

Group health education is one approach to medication problems. Education can help to *create* positive health behaviors; early intervention of another kind is often needed to *correct* negative behavior. A drug awareness center for the elderly—including consumer and professional education, a drug information hot line, medication counseling, crisis intervention, and health referral and follow-up—could provide a more comprehensive program. This is not a new idea. We are suggesting that the principles of drug education and counseling for young people be applied to an older age-group.

A drug awareness program is not designed to discourage or encourage drug use, but to stress the appropriate use of drugs when they are necessary. People over the age of sixty-five are a high-usage, high-risk group of drug consumers, and group health education can help them to more safely and effectively manage their medications. If professionals take an aggressive approach to consumer education, we can begin to eliminate the unnecessary complications of drug therapy.

REFERENCES

1. Brady, E. S.: Drugs and the elderly. In Davis, R. H. and Smith, W. K. (Eds.): *Drugs and the Elderly*. Los Angeles, Ethel Percy Andrus Gerontology Center, U of S Cal, 1973.
2. Brenner, J.: How to set up a health education program. *Joint Project on Staff Development for Services to the Aging*. Vol. 2. Urbana, Jane Addams School of Social Work, University of Illinois in cooperation with the Illinois Department on Aging, 1975.
3. DuPont, R.: Testimony before the Subcommittee on Aging and Subcommittee on Alcoholism and Narcotics of the U.S. Senate Committee on Labor and Public Welfare, Washington, D.C., June 7, 1976.
4. Gorrod, J. W.: Absorption, metabolism, and excretion of drugs in geriatric subjects. *Gerontol Clin, 16*:30-42, 1974.
5. Green, L. W.: The potential for health education includes cost effectiveness. *Hospitals, 50*:57-61, 1976.
6. Greenblatt, S.: *Social Aspects of the Use of Medication by the Elderly*. Paper presented to the Conference on Medication Use Among Older Adults, Augustana Hospital and Health Care Center, Chicago, April 2, 1976.
7. Hallberg, J. C.: The teaching of aged adults. *J Gerontol Nurs, 2*:13-19, 1976.
8. Hamm, B.: Paper presented to Drug Use and the Elderly: Perspectives and Issues Conference, National Institute on Drug Abuse, Rockville, Maryland, June 12-13, 1975.
9. Healy, K. M.: Does preoperative instruction really make a difference? *Am J Nurs, 68*:62-67, 1968.
10. Hecht, A.: The common cold: Relief but no cure. *FDA Consumer, 10*:4-9, 1976.
11. Isbister, J.: Testimony before the Subcommittee on Aging and Subcommittee on Alcoholism and Narcotics of the U.S. Senate Committee on Labor and Public Welfare, Washington, D.C., June 7, 1976.
12. Kayne, R. C.: Drugs and the aged. In Burnside, I. M. (Ed.): *Nursing and the Aged*. New York, McGraw-Hill, 1976.
13. Lasagna, L.: Drug effects as modified by aging. *J Chronic Dis, 3*:567-574, 1956.
14. Mintz, M.: The risk in drug ads. *Washington Post, 206*: (June 28, 1976).

15. Musser, R. D. and O'Neill, J. J.: *Pharmacology and Therapeutics.* New York, Macmillan, 1969.
16. Onek, J., Greenberger, M., and Ensminger, B.: *Petition to the FDA to Require More Adequate Patient Labeling of Prescription Drugs.* Consumers Union of the United States, Inc. and National Organization for Women, March 31, 1975.
17. *Physicians' Desk Reference.* Oradell, New Jersey, Medical Economics Company, 1976.
18. Roback, G. A. (Ed.): *Distribution of Physicians in the U.S., 1972.* Center for Health Services Research and Development, American Medical Association, 1972.
19. Schwab, M.: Caring for the aged. *Am J Nurs,* 73:2049-2053, 1973.
20. Schwartz, D., Wang, M., Zeitz, L., and Goss, M.: Medication errors made by elderly, chronically ill patients. *Am J Public Health,* 52:2018-2029, 1962.
21. Task Force on Prescription Drugs: *The Drug Users.* Washington, D.C., U.S. Govt Print Office, 1968.
22. U.S. Senate Subcommittee on Long-Term Care of the Special Committee on Aging: *Nursing Home Care in the United States: Failure in Public Policy. Introductory Report.* November, 1974.
23. Wake, C. D.: Attitudes of medical students toward the aged. *Geriatrics,* 24:58-59, 1969.

Chapter 13

COMMUNITY RESPONSIBILITY FOR DRUG USE BY THE ELDERLY

BARBARA P. PAYNE, PH.D.

IT HAS LONG BEEN recognized that the community has responsibility for control of the use of drugs. Drug problems are not new social problems, but the types of drug problems accompanying increased longevity and the growing number of older people are new.

The popular concept of drug misuse or abuse is that the drug problem is a youth problem about which society should do something. An equally popular concept is that drug abuse is limited to illegal or "recreational" drug use. So pervasive are these popular conceptions of the drug phenomenon that even the elderly, who proportionately receive more prescription drugs than any other age-group, appear to limit drug problems to teenagers and "the youth." Ross, Greenwald, and Linn[13] studied elderly people's perception of the drug scene and found that, although two-thirds of their elderly sample were taking some medication, they held the least favorable attitudes toward youthful drug users.

Other chapters in this volume analyze various facets of drug use and abuse by the elderly which destroy some of the popular misconceptions of this problem and identify the elderly drug scene as a new and serious social problem. This chapter, then, focuses on community responsibility for and response to this elderly drug problem.

DEFINITION OF COMMUNITY

In order to explore community responsibility for the problem, the delineation and definition of *community* must be determined.

Community is one of those ambiguous concepts one understands but has difficulty defining. Sociologists whose scientific interest includes the study of communities have attempted with limited success to reach agreement on a definition of community. For example, Hillery[10] identified over ninety different definitions or meanings of community. Writers in this area have used the term variously to designate a village, a neighborhood, a small town, a subarea of a city, an ethnic or racial group, an occupational-economic group, or any collection of people of like minds. The mass media (and television in particular) are contributing to the development of the concept of a national community which minimizes locality boundaries. A widely accepted definition of community and the one assumed in this chapter is that of Roland Warren:[16] "Community is that combination of social units and systems which perform the major social function having locality relevance.... These functions are: (1) Production—distribution —consumption; (2) Socialization; (3) Social control; (4) Social participation; and (5) Mutual support."

The problem of definition and geographical designation has been compounded by the impact of rapid urbanization on the structure and function of local communities, regardless of their size. Major changes impinging on communities demand a new formulation of the concept of community. Warren describes this reformulation as the "great change" that led to increased orientation of local community units and indeed the total community, toward extracommunity systems (other cities, the state, region, and nation) of which they are a part. The new community structure is a complex horizontal and vertical pattern of relationships. (Vertical patterns refer to extracommunity relations, while horizontal patterns refer to intracommunity relations.) Furthermore, Warren[16] notes that the vertical ties are not only stronger than the horizontal ties, but operate continually to strengthen the vertical ones.

The responsibility of a community for specific problems such as drug use and abuse is determined by these structures. The ability of local communities to solve or even to intervene in drug-related problems is limited by, and dependent on, the extracommunity (vertical) ties. Discussion, policies, and programs related to the problem are most frequently formulated outside the local community. The community as the local outlet operates these programs and implements the policies through local (horizontal) ties. However, it is easier to get agreement that a specific social condition is the community's responsibility than to determine who specifically in the community is to assume that responsibility.

Although a comprehensive analysis of community responsibility for drugs and the elderly normally employs a model encompassing both vertical and horizontal structures, this chapter deals only with the local community's efforts to take effective action and on those responses than can only be made in the local community where the individual old person lives and receives his drugs.

SOCIAL INFLUENCES ON ELDERLY DRUG ABUSE

Old age, unlike other stages in the life cycle, brings many social losses not related to personal failure but to societal insensitivity and neglect which impose severe if unobtrusive psychological stress on the elderly. The social loss older persons experience through retirement, death of a spouse or of close family members and friends, and loss of economic power contribute to stress, depression, isolation, and feelings of helplessness. Furthermore, these losses are, for the most part, irreversible. These sociopsychological conditions lead to physical complaints and psychological disturbances. As Rosow[12] points out, "People's mental health reflects not only their psychological state and the personality change within them but also events in the world around them—events that give pleasure, impose hardship and strain, create opportunities, make life easier or more exhilarating, and drive men to madness."

Sociopsychological conditions lead many older people to seek relief from their anguish either through medication prescribed by their doctors, through alcohol, or, for an increasing number, through suicide. Suicide is currently one of the ten leading causes of death in the United States for persons forty-five to sixty-four years of age, and the rate is highest for older white men, for widowers more than for widows.[15] Furthermore, it is estimated that one in three suicides is accomplished by a drug prescribed by a physician. Benson and Brodie[1] report that the major factors in suicidal attempts by old persons are chronic illness, social losses, insomnia, and depression, all of which are conditions that can be alleviated by prescriptions for hypnotic and therapeutic drugs. However, many of these drugs not only treat the condition but provide the older person with the access and familiarity with a convenient medium of suicide. This is in agreement with Benson and Brodie's opinion that the correlation between increasing insomnia associated with old age and the availability of barbiturates as a suicidal means is apparent.[1] Some barbiturates and psychotropic drugs may produce or intensify preexisting depressive and suicidal tendencies. If they are ingested with alcohol—which is also a depressant and easily obtained—the effects are potentiated. Davis and his associates[8] warn that as few as six tablets of secobarbitol (100 mg) taken with alcohol can cause death.

A new type of mental health problem, *nocturnal neurosis*, has been identified by Cohen[5] as being directly related to social factors. Nocturnal neurosis is characterized by a mixture of neurotic symptoms, including hypochondriasis, neurasthenia, insomnia, anxiety, and depression, which are either minimal or absent in the daytime. At night, however, these symptoms show a pronounced increase in both quantity and severity, especially in persons recently isolated due to the death of a spouse or close relative, moving, or retirement. Cohen[5] found that one-half of the elderly subjects in medical consultations in several midtown Manhattan facilities suffered from nocturnal neurosis.

It is speculated by Cohen[5] and by Bourg[2] that significant urban social conditions contribute to this nocturnal discomfort. For example, not only do older persons fear burglars at home, but they are also intimidated by the hassles of city (and suburban) night life, such as mugging and assault, which deter them from leaving home at night. Furthermore, it is assumed by family, neighbors, and most of the persons who provide services and programs for the elderly, e.g. senior centers, churches, and city recreational programs, that the elderly do not go out at night because they either do not want to, need their rest, or lack transportation (do not drive at night).

Neighbors are an important support system for most older people, and, according to Cantor's study,[4] most older people (about 80%) sit and talk together with neighbors in parks or open spaces. Cantor observes that "daytime programs and activities in lounge areas of agencies or centers often are superfluous or have a meager impact since most of the elderly are already interacting satisfactorily during the day."[4] At night, this neighborhood support is withdrawn. A survey of agencies in Manhattan has revealed that few have evening programs which are geared to their clientele.[5] One of the major radio stations in Atlanta with a 12 PM to 5 AM call-in program reports that many of their calls are from older persons who are lonely—and awake at these hours.

Rosow[12] has identified five specific social losses and their consequences that we believe contribute to the social sources of drug misuse by older people. They also provide a point of possible intervention by the community.

> First, the loss of roles excludes the aged from significant social participation and devalues them. . . .
> Second, old age is the first stage of life with systematic status loss for an entire cohort. . . .
> Third, persons in our society are not socialized to the fate of aging. . . .
> Fourth, because society does not specify an aged role, the lives of the elderly are socially unstructured. . . .
> Finally, role loss deprives people of their social identity.

Social losses are not treatable by pills. There is no pill to cure loneliness, boredom, or grief over the loss of a beloved one. The effects of social loss can be relieved through a variety of socially structured events and access to participation. Many psychological and physical conditions, however, can be improved by physical and social programs rather than by drugs, thus reducing the hazards of drug misuse or side effects.

COMMUNITY RESPONSES TO ELDERLY DRUG USE

In the review of the social factors influencing drug use, it has become evident that the drug problems of older persons cannot be separated from social, physical, and psychological stresses accompanying old age. One of the first responses the community needs to make is to become sensitive to the conditions that create the tendency to misuse drugs. This requires attention to general attitudes toward the elderly and to the specific areas where we have been insensitive.

In addition to the need for such sensitivity among physicians and pharmacists, educational campaigns to promote awareness of drug misuse among the aging themselves ought to be developed and supported by public and private groups, including professional groups, educational institutions, and the mass media. Brady, addressing the responsibility of social workers and service delivery persons in local communities, recommends:[3]

> We must become educators or—in a very real sense—missionaries, bringing the gospel of rational drug use to those areas of darkness where drug mis-adventures still occur. In situations where the elderly need advice, we must advise them, and wisely. Where they need our intervention, we must intervene, gently but positively. And if this intervention involves firm consultation with those who contribute to drug problems, we must have the courage to speak out on behalf of the patient.

In addition to increased sensitivity, the community must develop new social arrangements—programs and support systems—as nonchemical, positive alternatives to help older people reduce their dependence on, and overuse of, drugs. Several such programs and activities are discussed below.

Physical Exercise

Simple, nonexpensive exercise that can be done alone or with others, in the house or outside induces better sleep than medication and increases psychological feelings of well-being better than tranquilizers or alcohol. The simplest such exercise is walking. Nocturnal walks are being organized by residents in many apartment complexes and neighborhoods; these provide companionship, safety, and night activity to counteract nocturnal neurosis. Many articles and paperback books on exercise are in local bookstores, one of the most helpful of which for the elderly is that of deVries, *Vigor Regained*.[9]

Yoga is becoming popular with many older people. Classes

are offered in neighborhood senior centers, by the YMCA and YWCA, and in adult education programs presented by colleges and universities. There are also some television instructional programs, so that one can learn at home. In some areas, the YMCA and YWCA are offering special tennis and swimming classes for older people and are also reserving swim times for the elderly. Swimming, like walking, is one of the best and most therapeutic exercises, especially for the elderly.

Nutrition

Since one of the side effects of the use of drugs is a depressed appetite, adequate diets become very important. Studies of the dietary needs of older persons indicate the need for increased amounts of protein, less carbohydrates (especially sugar), more vitamin C in fruits, more iron in vegetables, and bulk in the form of bran and wheat breads. Less calories are needed, but a balanced diet is especially important to provide physical and psychic energy. A proper diet provides the basic psychological support to become socially active which, in turn, reduces isolation, boredom, and depression.

Night Activities

To deal with the conditions which lead to nocturnal neurosis, Cohen suggests the following social alternatives:[5]

- A. *Evening activities at a hotel.* Many hotels have a larger number of elderly people, and the staff members are able to arrange evening activity groups on the site. . . .
- B. *A dining-out club.* A staff member accompanies the elderly tenants to inexpensive restaurants. . . .
- C. *Evening programs at a senior citizen center.* At one midtown Manhattan center, a Wednesday Night Supper Club has been organized for 10 members, many of whom rarely go out in the evening. A taxi service is provided to take the participants home. . . .
- D. *Group outings.* In several centers, elderly persons are encouraged to meet in the evenings for dinner, to attend movies, or to play cards. . . .
- E. *Evening telephone liaison.* Many midtown Manhattan elderly do not view the telephone as an instrument for augmenting

social relationships, but see it as something to be used for emergencies or family crises. This is partly due to the relatively high cost (30 cents per call in a hotel). . . . We have begun to explore alternative uses of the telephone and have encouraged the residents to exchange telephone numbers.

Any of these nighttime activities could be organized by church groups, National Retired Teachers Association-American Association of Retired Persons chapters, civic clubs, sororities, or fraternities.

Community Volunteer Programs

Nonmedical community institutions have a partnership role in the health education and maintenance of older people. Neighborhood senior centers organized by churches, voluntary agencies, or local public agencies are usually more accessible than health facilities for elderly residents. While leaving to health centers the responsibility for diagnosis and treatment, there is a need for senior centers to provide new kinds of support systems comprised of caring and helping people which enable the elderly to live with purpose and meaning. One example of a new kind of community senior center is the Shepherd's Center, an ecumenical project involving twenty-two churches and synagogues in the Country Club-Waldo area of Kansas City. Elbert Cole, who has developed the program, describes it as a neighborhood response to the needs of older people and states that the general purpose of the Center is to "sustain older people in their homes and engage them in meaningful activities which gives purpose to life."[6] The older people in the community participate in both the planning and operation of the Center and state their specific objectives:[14]

> (1) To sustain the desire for independence characteristic of most elderly people, (2) to offer an integrative approach in meeting individual needs by bringing a wide variety of services from one center, (3) to focus on the elderly in a specific geographical area, small enough to accomplish the goals of the Center, (4) to provide opportunities for the elderly to serve and engage in meaningful activities, (5) to avoid isolating the elderly from the rest of the community, (6) to develop a model which could be duplicated elsewhere in the city and in other communities, (7) to make effective

use of existing community resources and programs designed to help those 65 and over.

To accomplish these goals, volunteers—most of whom are elderly themselves—provide the following services:[14]

Meals-on-Wheels. Men volunteers—and this is a "men's only" project—deliver a hot noontime meal five days a week to homebound persons or to persons temporarily limited after hospitalization or during an illness. Special diets are available when ordered by a physician. . . .

Shoppers. Older recipients in the target area unable to shop for themselves are taken to the market and other stores, or shopping is done for them.

Wheels That Care. By calling the transportation service, persons in the target area will be taken to medical facilities by volunteer drivers.

Handyman. Retired, skilled workmen make small repairs such as electrical, minor plumbing and carpentry—even painting—for a small fee. It is paid directly to the handyman.

Friendly Visitors. Many homebound persons receive regular visits and telephone calls from individuals through community organizations.

Companion Aides. Persons needing help with meals, housekeeping, and other chores may call the companion aide service. Rates are negotiable and paid to the employee.

Security and Protection. Crime prevention aides are able to offer information on home security and personal protection.

Care Twenty. Free meals and homemaker services are available to persons with limited income.

Night Team. The Shepherd's Center keeps in touch with people through a 24-hour answering service. The night team of clergymen responds to emergencies.

Health Enrichment Center. The Health Enrichment Center explores ways to assist participants in maintaining their health. Health lectures, exercise and nutrition classes are offered. Each Friday, nurses give health assistance and blood pressure tests. The annual Health Alert makes a variety of tests available without charge to persons 60 years of age and older. . . .

Life Enrichment Center. The Life Enrichment Center is a program bringing together those who have led fruitful lives until losing a loved one or being subjected to some other traumatic change. A clinical psychologist lectures and directs group participation and sharing. . . .

Adventures in Learning. Adult education classes and activities that feature a noon luncheon-forum. Some 400 older adults participate each week throughout the year.

New centers like the Shepherd's Center combine providing services and programming for the elderly with the development of new social roles that counteract some of the negative aspects of social aging. The Shepherd's Center volunteers, like the R.S.V.P. volunteers, Foster Grandparents, and other agency volunteer positions designed especially for the elderly, are performing new, valued social roles which, as Payne[11] has noted, provide continuity and maintenance of several role skills as well as development of new skills. Other groups providing experiences to aid persons with special needs are offered in most universities. Other public and private organizations are the Widowed Persons Service, stroke groups, and classes on assertiveness training. Older persons should be encouraged to participate in these groups (open to adults of any age).

Adult Day Care

In addition to activities for the well or functionally well elderly, communities are responding with the organization of day rehabilitation centers for those less active or moderately dysfunctional elderly who need limited treatment but cannot be left alone during the daytime. Such centers do not just provide a "sitter" service but administer medications for those who should not be responsible for their own medication and structure the time at the center with recommended physical and occupational therapy and social interaction.

Adult Education

Many new educational opportunities are available to the elderly through community colleges, universities, and adult-education courses. It is estimated that over half of the states have some tuition-free education program for the elderly, and many states provide full tuition to those over the age of sixty to attend state colleges. Some offer educational programs designed especially for the older student. For example, Fordham's College at Sixty, "... launched in 1973, is a unique educational program specifically designed to serve as a bridge between work and a return to or entry into academic life for retired and preretired adults. The program offers six seminars in such areas as psychology, philosophy, and science, each carrying two credits."[7] A certificate is awarded upon successful completion of four seminars. The certificate entitles these older students to enter the Liberal Arts College of Fordham without additional admission requirements.[7]

The organization of senior centers and the establishment of social programs and educational opportunities by communities must be accompanied by specific efforts to encourage older persons to participate and to offer positive reinforcement for those who do. Publicizing the events and their locations and ensuring easy access must also be a part of these community efforts to respond with social alternatives to the conditions that foster drug use.

SUMMARY

Community response to elderly drug use and abuse have included the following suggestions for action by both community organizations and the elderly themselves:

- Develop and sponsor educational campaigns to promote public awareness of the hazards of drug misuse especially among the elderly themselves
- Encourage existing public agencies and private organizations to provide nighttime and weekend activities to counteract nocturnal neurosis
- Sponsor and organize more neighborhood centers for the elderly that provide health maintenance programs, new social roles, and continuing educational opportunities
- Encourage the development by day care centers for the elderly by private and public agencies
- Support—and lobby for—free tuition in community colleges and universities for those over sixty.

Finally, the community can involve older people in the determination and the provision of the kinds of activities and life-styles that offer positive alternatives to an overreliance on drugs. Such action will undoubtedly result not only in new and meaningful community involvement for the elderly but also in an overall improvement in their health and well-being and a general reduction in the number of drug-related problems they will have.

REFERENCES

1. Benson, R. A. and Brodie, D. C.: Suicide by overdose of medicines among the aged. *J Am Geriatr Soc, 23*:304-308, 1975.
2. Bourg, C. J.: The elderly in a southern-metropolitan area. *Gerontologist, 15*:15-22, 1975.
3. Brady, E. S.: Drugs and the elderly. In Davis, R. H. and Smith, W. K. (Eds.): *Drugs and the Elderly*. Los Angeles, Ethel Percy Andrus Gerontology Center, U of S Cal, 1973.
4. Cantor, M. H.: Life space and the social support system of the inner-city elderly of New York. *Gerontologist, 15*:23-27, 1975.
5. Cohen, C. I.: Nocturnal neurosis of the elderly: Failure of agencies to cope with the problem. *J Am Geriatr Soc, 24*:86-88, 1976.
6. Cole, E.: Personal communication. July 31, 1977.
7. Comment: Special graduation. *Fordham*, 9:2, 1976.
8. Davis, J. M., Bartlett, E., and Termini, B.: Overdosage of psychotropic drugs: A review. Part I. Major and minor tranquilizers. *Dis Nerv Syst, 29*:157-164, 1968.
9. deVries, H. A.: *Vigor Regained*. Englewood Cliffs, New Jersey, Prentice-Hall, 1974.
10. Hillery, G. A., Jr.: Definitions of community: Areas of agreement. *Rural Sociol, 20*:111-123, 1955.
11. Payne, B. P.: The older volunteer: Social role continuity and development. *Gerontologist, 17*:355-361, 1977.
12. Rosow, I.: The social context of the aging self. *Gerontologist, 13*:82-87, 1973.
13. Ross, B., Greenwald, S., and Linn, M.: The elderly's perception of the drug scene. *Gerontologist, 13*:368-371, 1973.
14. *The Shepherd's Center*. Unpublished document. Kansas City, Missouri, The Shepherd's Center, 1973.
15. Suicide patterns in the elderly. *Geriatrics, 22*:68, 1967.
16. Warren, R.: *The Community in America*, 2nd ed. Chicago, Rand-McNally, 1971.

Chapter 14

DRUGS, AGING, AND SOCIAL POLICY

Frank J. Whittington, Ph.D.

THE PROBLEMS OLDER people encounter in the course of receiving and taking their drugs have been well documented by the other contributors to this volume. The reality and seriousness of these problems are certainly now beyond question. What remains is a discussion of the ways in which public policy has systematically helped to create, sustain, and exacerbate drug misuse both *by* and *of** the elderly.

A discussion of public policy on drugs and the elderly requires a few prefatory remarks about social policy in general. Policy, as a statement of general principle or philosophy which guides specific acts, is the lifeblood of the large, complex bureaucracies so necessary to urban, industrial society. Government is the largest and most complex of these bureaucracies and thus is the largest purveyor of policy, in this case, public policy, which is expressed either in law or in administrative rules or guidelines. But, as Gusfield notes, policy is determined both by the "agency" and the "act;" it is both the statement of general principle *and* ". . . the general pattern created by individual acts without reference to any directive statement."[33] Policy can be expressed either by what an organization says it does or by what its agents actually do. Public policy, therefore, encompasses not only the things which the government does in the name of its citizens but also the things—both known and unknown—government allows its citizens and institutions to do. If there is no policy prohibiting an action, then, in effect, the policy is to allow it.

To discuss social policies that produce or encourage drug

---

* My thanks to George Maddox (*see* Chap. 1) for this perceptive prepositional insight.

problems among the elderly, therefore, one must deal not only with law and government regulation but also with areas of behavior not yet regulated by government (or at least poorly regulated) and in which private organizations are allowed to set their own policies—policies which, although perfectly legal and proper from the organizational viewpoint, nevertheless may affect some members of society negatively. It is the thesis of this chapter that patterns of geriatric drug distribution and use, and thus misuse, depend largely on the policies of a number of powerful organizations and groups, including physicians, health institutions, and the drug industry. In addition, it is assumed that no one of these groups is wholly responsible for drug overuse and misuse by older persons, and that, as Bernstein and Lennard have pointed out, their very nature ". . . limits their competence to fully apprehend the far-reaching implications of the decisions they make, especially a full appreciation of the interpersonal, social and ecological costs of drug use."[5]

The primary aim of this chapter, then, is to examine each of these groups with respect to the role each plays in setting drug policy for older people, the problems each engenders for the elderly in the exercise of its role, and the relationship, if any, each bears to government and public policy. In addition, several general and specific proposals for new policies to help alleviate the problems are offered, and unanswered questions that suggest areas in which policy-relevant research is needed are raised.

Underlying institutional policies, however, is a firm cultural commitment to the scientific employment of chemical means (in fact, any means) in the battle against illness. That is, societal values, norms, and attitudes regarding drug use in general form a "cultural policy" that supports and guides many of the drug policies affecting the old. Such feelings and expectations almost certainly act as strong influences on the medical behavior of individual older patients, particularly in their interactions with various representatives of the medical care system who are, even apart from their medical orientations, subject to the effects of a drug-oriented society. Therefore, before proceeding to the discussion of the role of physicians, nursing homes, and the drug industry in setting drug policy for the elderly, it is helpful to consider American society's "cultural policy" toward drugs.

THE CULTURAL BASIS OF DRUG USE IN AMERICA

Man has always sought relief from his discomforts through chemical means. Blum and his associates surveyed 247 different nonliterate societies and found only 4 which did not employ any psychoactive (mood-altering) substance.[7] It was once observed by the famous physician, Sir William Osler, that "man has an inborn craving for medicine. . . . The desire to take medicine is one feature which distinguishes man, the animal, from his fellow creatures."[52] Nor have Americans been exceptional in this regard, as the social historian, de Tocqueville, noted in the 1830s: "In America, the passion for physical well-being is not always exclusive, but it is general; and if all do not feel it in the same manner, yet it is felt by all. The effort to satisfy even the least wants of the body and to provide the little conveniences of life is uppermost in every mind."[25] Present-day Americans are, it seems, no less concerned with "feeling good" than their ancestors; the difference is that the means to achieve such a state now exists.

Pharmacologists have produced remarkable results in the effort to defeat and control disease and malfunction. They have not only discovered drugs that act on the body's circulatory, pulmonary, digestive, and excretory systems and drugs such as penicillin which attack foreign organisms in the body, but they have produced a class of drugs, *psychoactives*, which act directly on the central nervous system. Psychoactives are mood-changing drugs which, when taken for medical reasons, are termed *psychotherapeutic*, because their primary purpose is to relieve some sort of psychic distress. The perfect psychoactive, if it could be produced, would be comparable to the mythical drug *soma*,* which Huxley describes in his futuristic novel, *Brave New World*, as "euphoric narcotic, pleasantly hallucinant," possessing "all the advantages of Christianity and alcohol; none of their defects."[35] Yet, present-day psychoactives are far from perfect; they have the effect, according to Bernstein and Lennard, of ". . . altering the clarity and capacity of all the senses—taste, touch, sight, hearing, and smell. Moreover, they diminish an individual's capacity to feel and control his own body, especially denying

---

* There is, by the way, now on the market a minor tranquilizer of the same name, which is marketed by Wallace Laboratories.

him access to sensual and sexual feelings."[5] Imperfection, however, has done little to slow either the production or use of such drugs. It is estimated that, in 1971, 230 million prescriptions for psychoactive drugs were written for noninstitutionalized persons in the United States (over one per person),[5] and that the American pharmaceutical industry annually produces billions of doses of tranquilizers, barbiturates, and amphetamines.[31] It appears that the national belief in "better living through chemistry" has ushered in what deRopp described in 1957 as "the chemopsychiatric era."[24] That is, Americans not only *believe* in drugs as a curative for all sorts of problems, we *value* them and their effects. We are afflicted with a new malady which might be termed *chemophilia*—the love of drugs. While generations reared and educated in the chemical age may have a more virulent case of the "illness," it also seems widespread among the elderly whose need for chemotherapy is usually greater.

Susceptibility to chemical comforts arises from several factors. First, Americans are generally in awe of science. They believe fervently in the ability of science to deliver the ultimate cure for all physical and social ills, and, while its record thus far is not flawless, it is astounding enough to have elicited an almost continuous reaffirmation of faith. Related to this attitude is the widespread belief in the near infallibility of the physician. In addition to being invested with the gift of healing, the doctor is also a scientist—if he prescribes a drug, most people never doubt that it is the correct one, in the proper dosage, applied at the appropriate time.

Another possible explanation for the willingness to medicate is the cultural reliance on the mass communications media for ideas and information. According to Barcus and Jankowski, "In a real sense, the mass media are the 'agenda-setters' of our culture. The selection of issues and the focus of attention that is given different aspects of society establish priorities for social action. . . . They tell us (1) what is; (2) what or who is important; (3) what is right or wrong; and (4) what is related to what."[1] If drug advertising in the media portrays drugs as the solution to most problems, if drugs are presented in the best possible light and their use is strongly encouraged, while the media, bound by self-interest, do relatively little to inform the public of their negative aspects, then it should come as no surprise if most people believe that their problems—from major infection to minor psychic distress and cosmetic imperfection—can be solved by taking a pill.

Perhaps in the final analysis, Americans *want* to believe that problems can be alleviated by such a neat, fast, painless method. So, they spend billions of dollars yearly on prescription and over-the-counter drugs and billions more on various kinds of useless medical quackery which promise no more than do legitimate pharmaceutical manufacturers—health, success, and long life. But such desires are evidently not limited to the present day, for, as McGlothlin states, "One of the consistent historical observations about drug using behavior is that excessive use flourishes during periods of social upheaval."[45] Although such abuse is certainly due to the social disorganization and personal alienation brought about by wars, migrations, and economic bad fortune, it also seems likely that the wish to narcotize oneself against such major catastrophes and the habit of whisking away life's minor ones with a tranquilizer are somehow related.

In fairness, it must be noted that the view of American society as vastly overmedicated is not universally shared. Mellinger and his associates surveyed the drug-taking habits of a broadly representative national sample and concluded that their findings failed to support an overmedication hypothesis.[47] In fact, they cite what Klerman has called "pharmacological Calvinism"[42] as one strong cluster of values which tend to reduce drug use in this society. These are the beliefs ". . . that use of psychotherapeutic drugs reflects personal weakness and undermines values traditionally placed on self-reliance, self-control, and will power to cope with one's problems."[47] There is no doubt that such beliefs do exist in this country and that they probably tend to reduce the overall level of drug consumption somewhat, but such beliefs are certainly not strongly held by most Americans, and there is little, if any, evidence that they exert a marked influence on the cultural habits of taking drugs to solve or control problems. The Mellinger data are extremely interesting, but they fail to undermine in a significant way the consistent findings of many researchers and reports of many clinicians (cited elsewhere in this volume) that too many drugs are prescribed, too many bought, and too many taken. The discussion now turns to an examination of the general drug policies or habits of the groups in question—physicians, nursing homes, and the drug industry—as they affect the elderly.

DRUGS, AGING, AND THE PHYSICIAN

Most of the drug problems experienced by older people arise from the doctor-patient relationship. Some of the problems are certainly caused by the patient, but many are the fault of the physician, or at least of his inadequate training in pharmacology and geriatrics. Nevertheless, over the past twenty or thirty years physicians have come to rely more and more on drugs as their primary mode of therapy. This is due largely to the pharmacological revolution and to the consequent increased emphasis on drug therapies in medical schools. However, the trend of increased prescribing of drugs has not often been accompanied by equal increases in pharmacological training, and geriatric pharmacology has probably been most seriously neglected.[57] Yet, this gap in the doctor's education is only part of a larger void—that created by the lack of serious geriatric medical training. While the elderly have disproportionately higher rates of illness and, thus, a greater need for medical care, attention to those needs in medical schools is practically nonexistent.

A recent survey of eighty-seven medical schools conducted by Senator Charles Percy of Illinois revealed that only three offered specialized training in geriatric medicine, and only seven more were planning to institute such courses of study in the future.[55] It is not surprising, then, that the American Medical Association reports over 18,000 pediatricians in practice in this country and only about 300 physicians who identify themselves as geriatricians.[18]

These gloomy statistics result primarily from three facts. First, physicians, including those in training, those in teaching, and those in practice, hold most of the same negative stereotypes toward old age and the elderly as do members of the larger society. Second, there is a general tendency to confuse the disease and aging processes by attributing disease-related (and sometimes drug-induced) symptoms to old age, about which, in the prevailing view, nothing can or need be done. And, finally, most physicians, like most other people, need the psychic reward of achieving success—medically speaking, of effecting a cure. The elderly, however, afflicted primarily with chronic illnesses, hold out little promise of such success and thus offer little incentive to the average physician to specialize in their care. For these reasons, doctors are disinclined to specialize in geriatric medicine or even to want to treat older patients, and, when they must, they are likely to misperceive the problem, to be anxious to "do something," and so to prescribe some medication, often a psychoactive drug, in an effort to ease the pain all around.

Moreover, physicians have fostered the growing tendency to "medicalize" all aspects of life; that is, as Bernstein and Lennard state, "The theory used to recruit physicians and deploy chemical technology in the war against social deviance, crime, misbehavior, alcoholism, mental illness, drug-addiction, overanxiety, overweight, overindulgence, overactivity, underactivity, insomnia, overpopulation, sadness, rage, and bizarre ideas, derives from the determination that these conditions are analogous to medical problems and therefore can be solved through medical means."[5] The physician, then, is more often called upon to treat with drugs physical and psychic symptoms produced by everyday stresses and problems in living. That he is particularly willing to do so for the elderly is further evidence of his confusion of the social and physical aspects of aging.

As Bourne has noted, doctors ". . . frequently fail to consider the abuse potential in prescribing these drugs for the elderly, whereas, in contrast, in recent years they have become acutely aware of this issue in dealing with younger people."[8] This casual attitude toward the older drug abuser is perhaps best epitomized by the appalling and callous statement Townsend attributes to a California physician who was told that an older female patient was addicted to Percodan (an analgesic): "She's an old lady, let her enjoy it."[68]

Moreover, the heavy reliance on drug therapy, coupled with a general lack of detailed knowledge about contraindications, side effects, and drug interactions, particularly in the elderly, means that the busy physician tends to rely heavily on drug company literature, advertising, and "detail men" (salesmen) for his information. This is an unfortunate situation, since drug manufacturers are in business to sell drugs, not to educate doctors, and consequently the drug information they publish and distribute is often calculated to emphasize the likely benefits of the drug and to minimize the potential dangers. More will be said about drug companies later.

The physician is often not prepared to diagnose correctly the older patient's problems or to prescribe properly for them. As noted earlier, however, the older patient is not free of responsibility for the negative outcomes of drug therapy. The elderly, like younger patients, often have unrealistically high expectations of the physician and want him to "do something" to relieve the immediate problem, even if little can be done to effect a long-range cure.

Some patients arrive in the doctor's office having already self-diagnosed and wanting only a medical confirmation, preferably in the form of a prescription, of what they already "know." Many patients feel the need to receive something tangible in return for their money; others desire to be given something to "do" in order to get well, such as taking medicine. Such an order helps to confirm the patient in his social role of "sick person." According to the "sick role" notion, originally described by Parsons, to be relieved of normal responsibilities the sick person must, among other things, seek competent medical care and follow medical advice in order to get well.[54] Taking medication is one obvious sign that the patient is fulfilling his role obligations.

Finally, some patients, like the Biblical character Naaman (2 Kings 5:1-27), prefer that the prescription fit their own definition of good therapy. It may be true that "medicine doesn't have to taste bad to be good," but few patients welcome any drug that cannot be called "strong medicine." In many cases such as these, the patient goes from doctor to doctor until he finds one who is agreeable and prescribes the drug he wants. Physicians must contend not only with such self-directed patients but also (and particularly so for elderly patients) with families and institutional staffs, both of whom often demand "help" in the form of drugs in managing difficult situations, especially if the condition is chronic.

Another way in which the older patient may undermine the physician's best intentions is to fail to comply with his orders for the use of the medication. This is a common problem among the elderly and one with potentially disastrous results. Although one survey of physicians revealed that 51 percent felt that the age of their patients was unrelated to their compliance with instructions,[22] most other studies of compliance patterns have found the elderly to be particularly prone to noncompliance.[9, 10, 61] For example, Brand and his associates found that, while only about one-fourth (26%) of the forty- to forty-nine-year-olds in their sample failed to comply with doctor's orders, nearly one-half (46%) of those aged seventy to seventy-nine and more than 62 percent of those eighty and over were not following instructions.[10] Other factors, such as low income, low level of education, being unmarried, and multiple prescriptions—all characteristics typical of the elderly—also predisposed toward noncompliance. Significantly, the cost of drugs was by far the most often cited reason for the patient's failure to comply; 34 percent indicated that they either could not afford to buy the drugs the doctor had prescribed or could not afford to take them as often as he had ordered.[10] This suggests that undermedication may be a more troublesome problem among low-income, noninstitutionalized elderly than overmedication.

DRUGS AND THE NURSING HOME

Another group of drug problems plague the elderly in long-term care institutions. Although it is constantly noted in the gerontological literature that only 4 or 5 percent of the older population are institutionalized, this statistic only reflects the situation at any one time. The fact is often overlooked that one's actual *chance* of being institutionalized in this country is about one in four; that is, approximately 25 percent of the older population eventually end up in a nursing home or mental institution.[39, 53] Thus, nursing homes, which today receive the vast majority of the medically and mentally incompetent elderly who must be institutionalized, are facilities of immense importance within the medical care system. Unfortunately, neither the quality of care which many render to their patients nor the quality of governmental determination to monitor that care and punish abuses appears to reflect this importance.

Increasingly, however, from a variety of sources is coming evidence of substantial abuse—both therapeutic and economic—within nursing homes, and one of the most widely reported of such abuses, encompassing the administrative as well as the medical aspects of care, is that of the misuse of drugs. This misuse has been reported to occur in four possible ways: (1) overmedication; (2) undermedication; (3) misadministration; and (4) unauthorized or potentially dangerous drug experimentation. Since these problems are dealt with specifically elsewhere in this volume, only a brief summary is given here.

Overmedication of patients is perhaps the most often mentioned and serious form of misuse.[50, 68] It includes both cases in which a physician prescribes too many drugs or too powerful a drug (often a major tranquilizer) and cases in which drugs are administered by staff in doses that exceed either the amount prescribed or that needed.[69] Undermedication occurs most often in institutional settings when prescribed doses are either negligently or intentionally not administered by the staff or, in the case of intermediate care patients who are allowed to administer their own medications, when the patient fails to comply with medication instructions. This is just one of several types of medication errors that can occur, however. Others include patients being given the wrong drug, or a wrong dose, or having it administered by a wrong route or at the wrong time.[70] Estimates of such errors range from a low of 22 percent[40] to a high of 50 percent[21] of all administered doses. Finally, Townsend has described the sort of patient abuse that can occur when nursing homes cooperate with drug companies in the testing of experimental drugs on their patients, particularly when the patient is not fully competent to render "informed consent" and has no family members to safeguard his interests.[68]

Certainly, there are many nursing homes in which such abuses are not allowed or at least are rare. And, while there is much disagreement over just how common drug problems are in nursing homes, there is little concerning the major causes. First, as Elaine Brody has phrased it, there is a "greed for drugs" among many of the elderly who enter nursing homes.[11] They are in the habit of taking drugs, and, whether the habit reflects physical or psychological dependence, the prospect of having the drugs withdrawn is a frightening one. So, many who are institutionalized place great demands on physician and staff not to discontinue current medication and even to add new drugs.

A second and probably the most widely cited precipitating reason for drug overuse in nursing homes is the desire on the part of the staff to control the patients more easily.[48, 50, 66, 68, 70] This desire is reflected by the facts that tranquilizers constitute nearly 20 percent of all drugs administered in this country's nursing homes, and the two strongest such drugs—Thorazine and Mellaril—accounted for over half of all tranquilizers prescribed.[69] The composite picture that emerges from many accounts is that of an overworked, underpaid, untrained, and often unsympathetic staff whose primary goal is not to render treatment but to keep order, maintain work schedules, and avoid patient demands. Paramount among the methods available for achieving these goals is that of drugs—usually either tranquilizers or sleeping pills. But such medications are certainly more for the benefit of the staff than that of the patient, as Pfeiffer illustrates by relating an often asked question and his response:

> "Don't you think it is better to give a senile person 'sleepers' at night?" My reply would be to ask, "Better for whom?" Is it better for the patient or better for the nurse to keep the patient asleep.... You are surely going to perpetuate the problem by giving someone with chronic brain syndrome sleeping medications on a regular basis. You are dealing with someone who has very little functioning brain left, and to additionally impair that brain function with hypnotics which affect the cerebral cortex, I think is not a good idea except for very acute situations. In fact, I think it is a lousy idea.[57]

It is, however, an idea whose time has come in most of the nursing homes in this country.

Even more disturbing than the existence of such attitudes is the fact that they often permeate the entire nursing home staff—both professional and nonprofessional—and are generally part of a larger context and pattern of patient abuse. As Stannard documents, however, such general abuse is usually dispensed by the nonprofessional aides and orderlies who have most of the direct contact with patients and who ". . . share a latent culture due to their lower social-class origins, which regards the use of force and aggression as a legitimate means of resolving conflicts."[66] The drugging of patients into compliance must nevertheless be supported at all levels: by the nurse, whose marginal position as both a medical professional and an administrator often leaves her in the quandry of choosing between good medical and good management policy; by the physician, whose overloaded work schedule either prevents regular monitoring of his nursing home patients or prompts "gang visits"[68] during which he may pay only cursory attention to the patient while routinely signing almost any order for psychoactive control medications the nursing staff deems appropriate; and, finally, by the nursing home administrator, who is ever alert to the costliness of a low staff-to-patient ratio and who knows that a tranquil patient is less demanding of staff time.

The last charge, relating the desire for patient control to the cost of providing care, leads into a consideration of the final reason for drug abuse of nursing home patients: the pursuit of profit rather than rehabilitation. In fact, Moss and Halamandaris have characterized a large portion of proprietary nursing home care as "services to the needy by the greedy."[50] While this characterization may be somewhat strong, it is only a small distance off the mark, and perhaps in no other area have nursing homes been found to be as consistently profitable as in the area of drugs. First of all, there are few inhouse pharmacies which might help to control the wanton distribution of drugs because, except for the largest homes, they are uneconomical (which is to say "not profitable enough"). In the larger homes, however, as Mendelson documents, they are among the most profitable of the "ancillary services."[48] But neither are smaller homes denied access to drug profits if they are willing, as many apparently are, to demand "kickbacks" from the local pharmacist in return for all the home's drug business. Moss and Halamandaris describe the standard technique employed in these terms: "The pharmacist presents with his drug deliveries an unitemized bill for prescriptions to the nursing home. The nursing home then 'bills' each individual patient, collecting from those who pay for their own drugs and sending the rest of the bills [for Medicare or Medicaid patients] along to the welfare department, which pays without scrutinizing it very carefully. The nursing home receives the state's check and keeps a certain percentage of it for 'handling,' services rendered, or whatever."[50]

The percentage kicked back is generally at least 25 percent and sometimes as high as 40 percent and can include, in addition to cash, supplying the home or its owners with credit, supplies, or paid vacations, "renting" some space in the home (which may turn out to be a closet), or buying advertising space at inflated rates in the nursing home's newsletter.[50] Although it is difficult to know how widespread this practice is, Mendelson and Hapgood point out, "Neither the GAO [General Accounting Office] nor any other investigating agency has looked at more than a small fraction of the records. Yet, if the pattern found so far is typical of the industry—and there is every reason to believe it is—then there are literally millions of frauds waiting to be uncovered."[49] No matter the extent, however, this sort of practice is a double fraud: It is a financial fraud upon both the patient who pays his own bills and the American citizen whose Social Security contributions support both the Medicare and, along with state tax money, Medicaid programs, and it is a therapeutic fraud upon the patient who may have to suffer a malign tranquility because neither the money nor the will is available for social and rehabilitative services.

Two additional policy-relevant issues surrounding drug use in nursing homes must be mentioned. First is that of the use of social drugs, such as beer and wine, for therapeutic purposes. As early as the mid-1960s long-term care institutions were experimenting with the use of beer and wine in group or "pub" settings to increase sociability and to reduce incontinence and the need for sedatives. It was even noted by Becker and Cesar that ". . . small quantities of alcohol may promote improved functioning of brain syndrome patients by stimulating vasodilation and increasing blood supply to the central nervous system."[3] Although the experience with this rather unorthodox therapy has tended to be positive, the results of some studies are mixed, and

Zimberg has even warned of the very real danger of iatrogenic alcoholism among patients who are encouraged to use this drug.[73] Nevertheless, alcohol therapy will likely find its way into the therapeutic repertoire of more and more nursing homes.

Another therapeutic problem which institutions face is that of the management of pain—both physical and psychological—often associated with terminal illness. Cancer, in particular, is a disease that can produce almost unbearable pain which may last for months as the dying person is kept alive by heroic medical means. Aside from the issue of euthanasia, there is some debate over how medical personnel should respond to such pain. One philosophical view holds that the human condition is intrinsically painful and that physical suffering is one way in which life tests and builds an individual's character. Donald Kent summarized this view in another context with the phrase, "A few fleas is good for a dog,"[41] presumably to remind him that he remains a dog. A related but different argument against the use of drugs to reduce the pain of the dying patient is that death is a crucial part of life and ought to be experienced consciously with senses clear and undulled by analgesics. Obviously, these positions are not widely held, and most physicians and patients readily accept and employ painkilling drugs, especially in the management of severe pain. The problem, then, becomes one of judging the severity of the pain, while the danger again lies in the overwillingness of doctors, nurses, and nursing home administrators to respond to patient demand for ever stronger drugs to treat trivial complaints.

DRUGS, AGING, AND THE DRUG INDUSTRY

At first glance it might appear that those who misuse, rather than those who manufacture and supply, drug products are primarily responsible for the ill effects of their misuse. And, certainly, patients, physicians, and nursing homes all share blame. However, the drug industry, including both pharmaceutical companies, which develop, manufacture, advertise, and wholesale the drugs, as well as pharmacists who sell them directly to the consumer, must also ultimately shoulder a portion of the responsibility. In fact, some students of the general drug problem in this country[16, 43] subscribe to what Douglas has aptly described as a conspiracy theory in which the drug companies reap immense profits through aggressive and questionable marketing tactics. Specifically, ". . . drug companies are seen as corrupting, or intimidating doctors into hiding bad effects of drugs and prescribing them to unsuspecting patients; the users are seen as the dupes of advertising; and the solution is found in turning the drug companies into public utilities."[26] While this view overlooks the existence, noted earlier, of ". . . a great and growing demand for psychoactive drugs, a deep and restless search for organically and synthetically induced peacefulness, intoxification and mysterious highs. . . ,"[26] it does include, as Douglas points out, some basic truths.

First, contrary to industry propaganda which claims the industry's "basic purpose" to be ". . . the search for, and the production and distribution of medicines to prevent, cure or alleviate disease throughout the world,"[56] the real goal of drug companies, like all businesses, is to make money. The development and "distribution," i.e. sale, of drugs which people need and want is the *means* to this end, not the end itself. In this regard, drug companies have been markedly successful. Although drug industry literature again portrays itself as positively altruistic in its efforts to provide the American consumer with the drugs he needs and wants at bargain basement prices, the fact is that drug companies are among the most profitable of United States corporations, with net yearly earnings which have been hovering around 19 percent since 1964. In comparison, the average United States manufacturing firm has recorded profits of only about 12 percent per year over this period.[29]

The battle for profits is joined in several ways. The first is to develop newer, better, and more widely applicable drugs than competitors. However, the development of new drugs is a long, slow, expensive process that is legally regulated by the federal Food and Drug Administration.* When a drug is finally market-

---

* Although several observers have been harshly critical of the way in which the FDA oversees drug manufacturers,[60] its regulatory mandate has grown far faster than its fiscal ability to perform its functions.[6] Moreover, even Burack and Fox, leading proponents of the conspiracy theory, give the FDA generally high marks and argue only that it needs more discretionary power, particularly in the area of judging *relative* drug efficacy.[16]

able, therefore, the company must really push it in order to maximize its return on investment before it is rendered obsolete either by newer substitutes[51] or by public opposition due to its own ill effects.[26] The chief method of achieving this goal is under the guise of physician education which is carried out through both advertising and the aggressive salesmanship of detail men. Garai has eloquently characterized this process:

> . . . approximately three-quarters of a billion dollars is spent every year by some sixty drug companies in order to reach, persuade, cajole, pamper, outwit and sell one of America's smallest markets— the 250,000 physicans. Direct mail, medical journal advertising, paramedical publications, closed-circuit television, canned radio, exhibits at conventions, samples, premiums, visits by detail men— these make up the mighty promotional weaponry the drug companies use to bombard their market. And it is not too much to say that perhaps no other group in the country is so insistently sought after, chased, wooed, pressured, and downright importuned as this small group of doctors who are the *de facto* wholesalers of the ethical drug business.[30]

This barrage, coupled with that leveled directly at the consumer over-the-counter market, nicely complements Americans' apparent socially induced craving for chemical cures, working to keep demand high. Garai summarizes the roles which drug advertising played in the successful introduction of tranquilizers: "Tranquilizers have become big business in the past eight years, a new national habit. They may or may not be superior to barbiturates or meaningfully different from them in clinical effect. We may someday learn the answers to these questions, or we may not. The matter is largely academic. Effective promotion, sustained promotion has carried the day. The physicians have been sold. So has the country."[30]

To compound the indictment, the charge is often made that much of drug advertising, which is monitored by the Federal Trade Commission rather than the Food and Drug Administration, is, at best, misleading and, at worst, patently false.[16, 27, 43] Although the situation has been improving, the emphasis in all American advertising has always been on freedom of speech and caveat emptor rather than consumer protection. Even in cases of obvious abuse when action is taken, the lag between first offense and final judgment is often dangerously long.

The direct effect on the elderly of drug advertising is debatable, although Wynne and Heller have theorized that the elderly may be more susceptible to its appeal because of their greater need for relief of both physical and emotional symptoms.[71] Moreover, Busse surveyed full-page drug ads in several issues of the *Journal of the American Medical Association* and found that, while 25 percent of the ads were for psychopharmacological agents, less than 10 percent of these made any mention whatsoever of the drugs' geriatric applications or limitations.[17] This is almost certainly due to the fact that the overwhelming majority of drug testing is carried out on young, healthy people with almost no attention whatsoever paid to the drug's effects on older persons, particularly those in generally poor health. When drug advertisements do focus on the older patient, they have been shown to portray him negatively and to reinforce popular stereotypes of older people as "aimless, apathetic, debilitated, disruptive, hypochondriac, insecure, . . . out of control, sluggish, seclusive, [and] temperamental."[65]

Not only do most advertisements minimize the real and potential dangers of the drugs they extol, but they have tended steadily to increase the number of nonmedical complaints with which the drugs may be expected to deal.[63] Lennard and his associates label such tactics *mystification* and charge that "the pharmaceutical industry is redefining and relabeling as medical problems calling for drug intervention a wide range of human behaviors which, in the past, have been viewed as falling within the bounds of normal trials and tribulations of human existence."[43] For example, many ads for geriatric psychoactive drugs promise relief from such "symptoms" as psychic tension, emotional distress, insomnia, apprehension, incommunicativeness, unwillingness to participate socially, uncooperativeness, unfriendliness, and disinterest.[70] Perhaps even more disturbing is the tendency of many companies to promote their tranquilizers as "especially suited to the nursing home patient" because of their benefits to "all concerned"—patient, family, staff, and nursing home.[70] In addition to relief of the patient's symptoms, the ads offer the staff a "less complaining," "less demanding," "less dependent," "more cooperative patient" who is "easier-to-manage."[70] The message to the nursing home owner and administrator is economic in nature and even less ambiguous: "1. Relief of symptoms means more amenable patient. 2. Less troublesome patient requires less nursing care."[70] Such "scientific" reasons for utilizing a specific medication dovetail nicely with the strong desire, noted earlier, of many nursing home staffs and owners for just this kind of assistance.

A final charge against drug companies concerns their unfortunate readiness, along with physicians, to abandon old medications whose ill effects have become known and controllable in favor of newer ones whose problems are not yet clearly understood. Douglas argues that both drug manufacturers and physicians act in this way to protect their reputations before a dubious public which may begin to resist the use of drugs which receive unfavorable publicity.[26] Chambers and his associates have described how this process worked in the case of one particularly problematic sedative, methaqualone.[19]

Community pharmacists apparently play little active role at present in fostering drug misuse among their older customers, for they are, in the case of prescription medications, merely following the physician's instructions and serving as conduits from the drug company to the patient. They may assume somewhat more responsibility in the area of over-the-counter preparations when their clients seek their advice on which remedy to buy, but, other than through participation with nursing homes in drug-kickback schemes, the community pharmacist is hardly implicated. And yet, the lack of active concern and monitoring in so strategic a position may be a crucial contributing factor to the overall problem. The modern pharmacist has apparently lost the very powerful position he once held as a member of the health care team, and the reasons are not altogether clear, although Mechanic has offered several interesting insights.[46] The point is that he could be serving as the primary gatekeeper and monitor of all sorts of drug problems to which the elderly are subject but he is not. He could, in addition, perform a central role in the area of health and drug education but, so far, has failed to assume such a role.

ELDERLY DRUG POLICY PROPOSALS

Already more proposals for change in public policy toward the elderly exist than can ever be adopted, and perhaps, as Robert Harris suggests, most should not be.[34] Nevertheless, it seems appropriate at this point to offer some suggestions, based on the preceding discussion, for new social policy on drugs and the elderly.

First, the elderly (like most Americans) need to be re-educated to a new view of drugs, one which emphasizes a healthy skepticism toward their "miracle" properties and fosters an appreciation of nonintrusive, nonchemical therapies. They must accept major responsibility for monitoring and controlling their own drug intake and must insist that physicians, nurses, pharmacists, and other health care professionals provide them with the medical and pharmacological information they need in order to do it. Such goals obviously require intensive drug and health education for the elderly, and prototype programs of this sort are already functioning in some parts of the country.[44, 58, 67] These should be duplicated elsewhere and operated either through local community aging programs, public health agencies, hospitals, nursing homes, or home health programs such as visiting nurses.

As Cheung[20] and others[12, 26] have suggested, a national reporting system is needed to monitor drug problems, including those of the elderly, and provide reliable data on the nature and extent of elderly drug problems coming to professional attention. Such a network could be modeled on the DAWN program initiated by the Bureau of Narcotics and Dangerous Drugs, which gathers information from drug abuse treatment programs and hospital emergency rooms but would additionally include hospital in-patient services, nursing homes, physicians, and community clinics.

A number of policy proposals can be made concerning the physicians who prescribe most of the drugs which older people take. First, physicians desperately need more and better training —both in medical school and throughout their practice—in pharmacology and in geriatrics. One hopeful sign is the fact, reported by Senator Charles Percy, that, although only ten medical schools had, or were developing, a speciality in geriatrics, thirty-five schools reported having programs that placed students or interns in a nursing home setting for clinical training.[55] The AMA should move rapidly to designate geriatrics as a recognized medical speciality in order to establish it as a credible and prestigious area of medical study and practice. In addition, the physician must be able continually to update his knowledge of geriatric pharmacology without depending on drug company detail men. Cheung has suggested a national communications network to disseminate information on drug side effects and interactions directly to the physician,[20] while Muller has proposed a "neutral detailing force," independent of the drug companies, to educate busy doctors.[51] Whatever model is selected, it is clear that physicians have a great need for more clear, concise, unbiased information about the drugs they prescribe for their patients.

The thrust of pharmacological education should be to persuade doctors to rely less on drugs and more on other kinds of therapy. For example, if an elderly patient's depression is judged to be due to some social loss he has experienced, it makes little sense for the doctor to seek a medical solution to what is essentially a social or psychological problem. A more rational approach would be to attack the *cause* of the depression by either suggesting a replacement role or referring the patient to an appropriate counselor or agency rather than to treat the symptom by prescribing an antidepressant drug. This approach, of course, requires the physician to devote additional time to patient education and counseling, but this investment undoubtedly pays off in healthier, less physician-dependent patients.

Another needed innovation is that of a national drug-utilization review system that would establish guidelines for drug prescribing and periodically review physicians' prescribing habits to see that they are not systematically deviating from good prescription practices.[20] Muller argues that such a review might carry strong economic incentives if reimbursement for drug charges under a national health insurance plan were dependent on the physician's utilization of drugs listed in an official formulary which would be "restricted to safe, effective, and reasonably priced drugs."[51] Brody suggests, moreover, that this sort of utilization review could be instituted under present Medicare and Medicaid programs and could yield a wealth of both quality control and epidemiological data.[12]

The widespread acceptance of Health Maintenance Organizations (HMOs) which provide prepaid, comprehensive medical care might also curtail drug problems among the elderly. Browdy argues that there is less overprescribing of drugs in HMOs, because the physician does not worry about the cost to the patient of follow-up visits.[15] He may thus be more inclined to let the disease or symptom follow its natural course rather than to attempt to prescribe unnecessary drugs just to please the patient and send him on his way. The physician, in addition, has an economic stake in the actual overall health and well-being of the patient and would presumably be more conservative in his use of potentially harmful drug therapies. Currently, however, most HMOs tend to accept only relatively healthy persons and exclude many older people who are chronically ill, even though Medicare does pay for medical care delivered through an HMO, and Brody has clearly shown that such care can be provided at a lower cost than through a standard fee-for-service situation.[14] He notes, however, that the HMO concept is only one of several potential models of delivering comprehensive health care to the elderly,[13] which are discussed later.

A second major group of policy proposals concerns elderly drug use in nursing homes. Perhaps the first action that needs to be taken is that government at all levels should begin vigorously to enforce the many laws and regulations already available to control both the therapeutic drug abuse of the patient and the economic abuse of federal and state health care programs for the elderly. More careful monitoring, for example, of the drug-utilization reviews required of nursing homes which participate in the Medicare and Medicaid programs would undoubtedly serve to upgrade drug prescription and distribution habits in such institutions.[37] Another regulation that needs to be more vigorously enforced is that requiring the nursing home to engage the services of a consulting pharmacist if it does not have an inhouse pharmacy. Related to this situation is an economic control measure proposed by the United States Senate Subcommittee on

Long-Term Care which would eliminate the nursing home as the middleman in Medicare and Medicaid drug reimbursement.[70] This would greatly limit the ability of institutions to demand and receive a kickback from pharmacists' profits and would certainly soon reduce the cost to government of providing drugs to older patients under these programs. It would also reduce the financial incentive *not* to have an inhouse pharmacy, thus encouraging the initiation of such needed services.

The Senate Subcommittee on Long-Term Care also strongly recommends that only licensed nursing personnel be allowed to dispense medications in nursing homes and that residential facilities be required to provide special training to all staff members who handle drugs.[70] Just as important may be the general and regular inservice training of all nursing home personnel in geriatrics and gerontology, especially if such training is coupled with a comprehensive effort to build a sense of professionalism among these personnel (particularly aides and orderlies), by increasing salaries and hiring more selectively.

There is no doubt that most nursing homes have drug distribution and monitoring systems that are woefully inadequate to insure against drug administration errors, but, as discussed elsewhere in this book, model systems now exist that can greatly reduce such errors and contribute significantly to overall patient well-being.

Nursing homes should continue and intensify their efforts to develop and refine social and psychological therapies, such as reality orientation and remotivation therapy, which deal with the causes of the older patient's problems, e.g. isolation, de-socialization, etc., rather than with results such as depression, insomnia, and agitation. Although such therapies are certainly not always successful, they are much less intrusive, debilitating, and dangerous than standard drug therapy. In addition, Barney advocates active involvement on the part of interested community members in the affairs of the nursing home, both as volunteers working in patient care and therapy and as monitors of the quality of care the home can provide its residents.[2] She suggests that there is a definite connection between the owner of the home being actively involved in local community affairs, community members performing ombudsman functions for the patients, and good quality care. Kane and his associates have even made the radical, yet eminently sensible, suggestion that Medicare and Medicaid reimbursement schedules be tied, not to the cost of maintaining a patient in bed for a day, but to the home's success in rehabilitating him.[38] They advocate replacing the present three-level system of classifying patients with a prognostic system and reimbursing the nursing home according to whether patients achieve prognosed levels of function. They also indicate that a team approach to providing patient care utilizing both medical and social service professionals was both therapeutic and cost-effective.[38]

Several recommendations can be made with respect to drug industry policies and elderly drug misuse. First, relatively little is known about geriatric pharmacology, particularly in the areas of proper dosage, likely adverse reactions, and possible effects of long-term drug therapy. For example, Johnson relates how, as a medical student, he learned "Young's Rule," by which infants' and children's doses of medicine are calculated but decries the lack of a parallel "Old's Rule" to accomplish the same task for older people.[36] Drug companies should also work on the development of safer drugs and not just more powerful ones. Douglas has prosed that "unless there is such an urgent need for it that a high degree of risk seems justified, government regulations should prevent the introduction of any new drug in any guise until its addictive effects are clear, until the nature of its withdrawal problems are clear, until its overdose effects are clear, and until medical methods of handling these problems are developed and made known to clinicians."[26] Moreover, as Burack and Fox have argued, the FDA should be allowed to determine relative efficacy and prohibit any new drug that does not improve upon the therapeutic ability of older drugs.[16] Further, it should be the responsibility of the drug manufacturers to design simplified means of medication dispensing, including containers which the elderly can easily handle and "reminder" devices, possibly similar to the birth-control pill disc, for memory-impaired older persons.

The Federal Trade Commission, charged with overseeing drug company advertising and promotion, should broaden and toughen its regulatory policies with respect to all drugs and particularly those most often used by older people. Of course, drug companies feel that they have the inherent right of any business to hawk their wares and even engage in a bit of harmless puffery, as is the habit of most other advertisers of consumer goods. Yet, drugs are not merely another brand of laundry detergent promising "whiter-than-white" results, and they are not sold by taste like cornflakes or candy bars. They are potentially toxic substances whose *only* purpose is supposed to be to save lives and relieve suffering. Since prescription drugs fall into a category called *ethical* drugs, it would seem logical that they ought to be promoted in a special manner as a consumer item. After all, it certainly would be considered unethical (by present standards) for a physician to advertise his services as superior in therapeutic or life-saving value to those of his fellow doctors. Even "tasteful" ads are now considered to be unethical, so why must drug companies be allowed such wide latitude in their claims? The answer, of course, is that they need not be. If the task of "educating" physicians were removed from the drug companies and given over to some independent, unbiased entity, similar to those described by Cheung[20] and Muller,[51] which could efficiently communicate current information on drug efficacy and safety to the physician, then ethical drugs might, in truth, be ethically distributed.

As noted above, the community pharmacist is not an active cause of drug problems among the elderly, but there is no reason he could not become an active agent of prevention of drug misuse. Muller,[51] Mechanic,[46] and others have pointed out the pharmacists' great potential for serving both as a monitor of drug-prescribing and drug-taking habits and as a patient counselor on drug and even general health matters. Wynne and Heller, for example, have described the way in which California pharmacists have cooperated with physicians in the operation of a computerized monitoring system which is designed to detect drug prescribing or dispensing abuses.[72] It has also been effective in reducing drug costs under the state's Medicaid program. Although many writers have noted the "incomplete professionalization"[23, 71] and economic motivation[28] of many pharmacists, the opportunity to assume once again an honored and necessary position among health care providers is certainly available.

Finally, it is proposed that major new efforts be undertaken to develop and extend community medical and social programs, such as home health care, adult day care, and community mental health programs, each including a drug monitoring and education component, and all of which are aimed at assisting the elderly to remain in their own homes and out of institutional settings for as long as they are able. While many older people have chronic conditions requiring some sort of care for an extended period, such care increasingly need not be provided within the walls of an institution, for, as Bell has cogently demonstrated, the phrase *long-term care* is clearly not synonymous with institutional care.[4] Thus, the well-known phrase *alternatives to institutionalization* must come to symbolize a wide range of sociomedical services designed to forestall, but not necessarily to eliminate, the need for institutionalization. Institutionalization is, after all, itself an alternative and often the final one;[64] thus, as we have argued, the goal of optimizing patient care in nursing homes is a worthy one. We must, however, be at least as committed to the provision of high quality care to the community-dwelling older person when the evidence indicates that he would fare better at home than in an institution.

A final and, indeed, crucial proposal is that intensive and broad-ranging research efforts be quickly undertaken in all areas and on all aspects of the elderly drug problem. The argument for such an omnibus approach can be made with confidence, because so little empirical data on the nature, extent, settings, and causes of drug use and misuse among the elderly presently exist that any addition to the knowledge in this area would be welcome.

Some researchable issues seem more immediately important than others. For example, while a great deal of clinical observation supports the notion that drugs are vastly overused in nursing homes, a number of observers feel that elderly in the community are more likely to undermedicate,[32, 59] primarily through noncompliance with physicians' orders and inability to afford prescribed medications.[10] However, so little is known about the drug-taking habits and compliance patterns of community elderly that such a position cannot now be supported. Another fertile area for research is the physician's relations with his elderly patients. It has throughout this chapter been argued on the basis of admittedly scanty evidence that physicians overprescribe drugs, particularly psychoactive drugs, for their older patients, especially those in nursing homes. Additional studies are needed of this important encounter, however, before such charges may be accepted with total confidence.

There is no empirical data on the cultural, social, or psychological bases for patients' misuse; that is, it is assumed, but not proven, that such variables as sex, race, age, education, occupation, religion, and personality factors may all have certain effects on drug misuse. Other promising areas of investigation include the elderly's susceptibility to drug company advertising of over-the-counter medicines, their use of such remedies, and the actual therapeutic benefit they receive from them; the reliance by older people on folk medicine, home remedies, and nostrums; the extent of employment of placebo therapy by physicians for community, as opposed to nursing home, residents and its judged effectiveness; and, for institutionalized elderly, the relative effectiveness of social and drug therapies, the attitudes of staff toward their patients and toward drugs, and the relationship between these attitudes and staff willingness to use drugs to maintain control of the patient.

Finally, it is imperative that research methodologies be devised to evaluate the effectiveness of the various drug education or control programs which have been mentioned and suggested. Only by judging their relative impact on the drug-taking habits of older people can it be decided whether to commit large amounts of money to their broad-scale implementation.

CONCLUSION

In sum, the issue of drug use and misuse among older people is so broad and so many-faceted that its policy dimensions can hardly be delineated in one chapter. Yet, an effort has been made to examine the central arenas of the problem, to discuss in some detail the therapeutic dramas being played out in those arenas, and to make general and specific suggestions for the kinds of changes in social policy which seem indicated. Doubtless, much has been inadvertently omitted, but what has been included is certainly sufficient to define an issue likely to command in the future an increasing share of the public attention. A former under-secretary of the Department of Health, Education and Welfare is quoted by Ryder as having said that, "Federal programs are fine if you are old enough, sick enough, or poor enough. If you aren't, you must wait until you are older, sicker, or poorer."[62] Let us hope that the problems associated with the misuse of drugs by older people do not have to wait until they get worse before new social policies are adopted to serve as guides for concerted remedial action.

REFERENCES

1. Barcus, F. E. and Jankowski, S. M.: Drugs and the mass media. *Ann Am Acad Pol Soc Sci, 417*:86-100, 1975.
2. Barney, J. L.: Community presence as a key to quality of life in nursing homes. *Am J Public Health, 64*:265-268, 1974.
3. Becker, P. W. and Cesar, J. A.: Use of beer in geriatric psychiatric patient groups. *Psychol Rep, 33*:182, 1973.
4. Bell, W. G.: *Policy and Practice in Long-Term Care of the Elderly: A Proposal for Change.* Paper presented to the Annual Meeting of the Gerontological Society, Portland, Oregon, October 28-November 1, 1974.
5. Bernstein, A. and Lennard, H. L.: Drugs, doctors and junkies. *Society, 10*:14-25, 1973.
6. Bitter pills for the FDA. *Newsweek, 90*:93, 95, July 18, 1977.
7. Blum, R. H. and Associates: *Society and Drugs.* San Francisco, Jossey-Bass, 1969.
8. Bourne, P. G.: Drug abuse in the aging. *Perspect Aging, 2*:18-20, 1973.
9. Brand, F. N. and Smith, R. T.: Medical care and compliance among the elderly after hospitalization. *Int J Aging Hum Dev, 5*:331-346, 1974.
10. Brand, F. N., Smith, R. T., and Brand, P. A.: Economic barriers in medical care as a factor in patients' non-compliance. *Public Health Rep, 91*:72-78, 1977.
11. Brody, E. M.: Quoted in National Institute on Drug Abuse: *Drug Use and the Elderly: Perspectives and Issues.* Proceedings of The Conference on Drug Use and the Elderly, National Institute on Drug Abuse, Rockville, Maryland, June 12-13, 1975.
12. Brody, S.: Quoted in National Institute on Drug Abuse: *Drug Use and the Elderly: Perspectives and Issues.* Proceedings of The Conference on Drug Use and the Elderly, National Institute on Drug Abuse, Rockville, Maryland, June 12-13, 1975.
13. Brody, S. J.: Evolving health delivery systems and older people. *Am J Public Health, 64*:245-248, 1974.

14. Brody, S. J.: Prepayment of medical services for the aged: An analysis. *Gerontologist, 11*:152-157, 1971.
15. Browdy, S.: HMO vs. fee-for-service: An insider's story. *Med Econ, 52*:71-74, 1975.
16. Burack, R. and Fox, F. J.: *The New Handbook of Prescription Drugs.* New York, Ballantine, 1975.
17. Busse, E. W.: Preface. In Eisdorfer, C. and Fann, W. E. (Eds.): *Psychopharmacology and Aging.* New York, Plenum Pr, 1973.
18. Carlson, J. R.: What are the prospects? Health in America. *Center Magazine, 5*:43-47, 1972.
19. Chambers, C. D., Bridge, T. P., Petersen, D. M., and Ellinwood, E. H.: Methaqualone: Another "safe" sedative? *J Drug Issues, 4*:126-129, 1974.
20. Cheung, A.: Quoted in National Institute on Drug Abuse: *Drug Use and the Elderly: Perspectives and Issues.* Proceedings of The Conference on Drug Use and the Elderly, National Institute on Drug Abuse, Rockville, Maryland, June 12-13, 1975.
21. Crawley, H. K., III, Eckel, F. M., and McLeod, D. C.: Comparison of a traditional and unit dose drug distribution system in a nursing home. *Drug Intell Clin Pharm, 5*:166-171, 1971.
22. Davis, M. S.: Variations in patients' compliance with doctors' orders: Analysis of congruence between survey responses and results of empirical investigations. *J Med Educ, 41*:1037-1048, 1966.
23. Denzin, N. K. and Mettlin, C. J.: Incomplete professionalization: The case of pharmacy. *Soc Forces, 46*:375-381, 1968.
24. deRopp, R. S.: *Drugs and the Mind.* New York, Grove, 1961.
25. de Tocqueville, A.: *Democracy in America.* Vol. 2. (H. Reeve, trans.) New York, Knopf, 1948.
26. Douglas, J. D.: Drug crisis intervention. *Drug Use in America: Problem in Perspective.* Vol. 4. The Technical Papers of the Second Report of the National Commission on Marijuana and Drug Abuse. Washington, D.C., U.S. Govt Print Office, 1973.
27. Dowling, H. F.: *Medicines for Man: The Development, Regulation, and Use of Prescription Drugs.* New York, Knopf, 1970.
28. Francke, D. E.: Let's separate pharmacies and drugstores. *Am J Pharm, 141*:161-176, 1969.
29. Fulda, T. R.: *Prescription Drug Data Summary: 1974.* Washington, D.C., Social Security Administration, U.S. Department of Health, Education and Welfare.
30. Garai, P. R.: Advertising and promotion of drugs. In Talalay, P. (Ed.): *Drugs in Our Society.* Baltimore, Johns Hopkins U Pr, 1964.
31. Graham, J. H.: Amphetamine politics on Capitol Hill. *Trans-action, 9*:14-22, 53, 1972.
32. Greenblatt, S.: *Social Aspects of the Use of Medication by the Elderly.* Paper presented to the Medication Use Among Older Adults Con-

ference, Augustana Hospital and Health Care Center, Chicago, April 2, 1976.
33. Gusfield, J. R.: The (f)utility of knowledge? The relation of social science to public policy toward drugs. *Ann Am Acad Pol Soc Sci, 417*:1-15, 1975.
34. Harris, R.: *Translating Ideas into Action: Structuring the Problems.* Paper presented to the Duke University Conference on Assessment and Evaluation Strategies in Aging: People, Populations and Programs. Asheville, North Carolina, May 19-21, 1977.
35. Huxley, A.: *Brave New World.* New York, Harper & Row, 1946.
36. Johnson, A. N.: The physician's role in the care of the aging. *Gerontologist, 10*:33-37, 1970.
37. Kabat, H. F., Kidder, S. W., Martilla, J. K., and Stewart, J. E.: *Drug Utilization Review in Skilled Nursing Facilities: A Manual System for Performing Sample Studies of Drug Utilization.* Washington, D.C., U.S. Department of Health, Education and Welfare, 1975.
38. Kane, R. L., Jorgensen, L. A., Teteberg, B., and Kuwahara, J.: *Is Good Nursing-home Care Feasible?* Paper presented to the Annual Meeting of the Gerontological Society, Portland, Oregon, October 28-November 1, 1974.
39. Kastenbaum, R. and Candy, S.: The four percent fallacy. *Int J Aging Hum Dev, 4*:15-21, 1973.
40. Kayne, R. C. and Cheung, A.: An application of clinical pharmacy in extended care facilities. In Davis, R. H. and Smith, W. K. (Eds.): *Drugs and the Elderly.* Los Angeles, Ethel Percy Andrus Gerontology Center, U of S Cal, 1973.
41. Kent, D. P.: Social policy and program considerations in planning for the aging. In Kent, D. P., Sherwood, S., and Kastenbaum, R. (Eds.): *Research, Planning and Action for the Elderly.* New York, Behavioral Pub, 1972.
42. Klerman, G. L.: Psychotropic hedonism vs. pharmacological Calvinism. *Hastings Center Rep, 2*:1-3, 1972.
43. Lennard, H. L., Epstein, L. J., Bernstein, A., and Ransom, D. C.: *Mystification and Drug Misuse.* San Francisco, Jossey-Bass, 1971.
44. Maultsby, M. C.: Decreasing prescription suicides or a behavioral approach to irrational fears and prescribing. *J Am Med Wom Assoc, 27*:416-419, 1972.
45. McGlothlin, W. H.: Introduction. *J Soc Issues, 27*:1-6, 1974.
46. Mechanic, D.: Social issues in the study of the pharmaceutical field. In Mechanic, D.: *Politics, Medicine, and Social Science.* New York, Wiley, 1974.
47. Mellinger, G. D., Balter, M. B., Parry, H. J., Manheimer, D. I., and Cisin, I. H.: An overview of psychotherapeutic drug use in the

United States. In Josephson, E. and Carroll, E. E. (Eds.): *Drug Use: Epidemiological and Sociological Approaches.* Washington, D.C., Hemisphere, 1974.
48. Mendelson, M. A.: *Tender Loving Greed.* New York, Vintage Books, 1974.
49. Mendelson, M. A. and Hapgood, D.: The political economy of nursing homes. *Ann Acad Pol Soc Sci, 415*:95-105, 1974.
50. Moss, F. E. and Halamandaris, V. J.: *Too Old, Too Sick, Too Bad.* Germantown, Maryland, Aspen Systems, 1977.
51. Muller, C.: The overmedicated society: Forces in the marketplace for medical care. *Science, 176*:488-492, 1972.
52. Osler, W.: Teaching and thinking: The two functions of a medical school. *Montreal Med J, 23*:561-572, 1894-1895.
53. Palmore, E.: Total chance of institutionalization among the aged. *Gerontologist, 16*:504-507, 1976.
54. Parsons, T.: *The Social System.* New York, Free Pr, 1951.
55. Percy, C. H.: Opening statement. Hearing on Medicine and Aging: An Assessment of Opportunities and Neglect. U.S. Senate Special Committee on Aging, New York, October 13, 1976.
56. Pharmaceutical Manufacturers Association: *Key Facts About the U.S. Prescription Drug Industry.* Washington, D.C., Pharmaceutical Manufacturers Association, 1974.
57. Pfeiffer, E.: Use of drugs which influence behavior in the elderly: Promises, pitfalls, and perspectives. In Davis, R. H. and Smith, W. K. (Eds.): *Drugs and the Elderly.* Los Angeles, Ethel Percy Andrus Gerontology Center, U of S Cal, 1973.
58. Plant, J.: Educating the elderly in safe medication use. *Hospitals, 51*:97-102, 1977.
59. Prien, R.: Quoted in National Institute on Drug Abuse: *Drug Use and the Elderly: Perspectives and Issues.* Proceedings of The Conference on Drug Use and the Elderly, National Institute on Drug Abuse, Rockville, Maryland, June 12-13, 1975.
60. Quinney, R.: *Criminology: Analysis and Critique of Crime in America.* Boston, Little, Brown & Co., 1975.
61. Rodstein, M.: Prevention of disability in the aged. *Geriatrics, 21*:193-196, 1966.
62. Ryder, C. F.: *Translating and Transmitting Knowledge about Assessment and Evaluation: What, Who, How—Long-Term Care.* Paper presented to The Duke University Conference on Assessment and Evaluation Strategies in Aging: People, Populations and Programs. Asheville, North Carolina, May 19-21, 1977.
63. Seidenberg, R.: Advertising and abuse of drugs. *N Engl J Med, 284*:789-790, 1971.
64. Shore, H.: What's new about alternatives? *Gerontologist, 14*:6-11, 1974.

65. Smith, M. C.: Portrayal of the elderly in prescription drug advertising: A pilot study. *Gerontologist, 16*:329-334, 1976.
66. Stannard, C.: Old folks and dirty work: The social conditions for patient abuse in a nursing home. *Soc Prob, 20*:329-342, 1973.
67. Subby, P.: *A Community Based Program for Chemically Dependent Elderly.* Paper presented to The North American Congress on Alcohol and Drug Problems, San Francisco, December, 1975.
68. Townsend, C.: *Old Age: The Last Segregation.* New York, Grossman, 1971.
69. U.S. General Accounting Office: *Drugs Provided to Elderly Persons in Nursing Homes Under the Medicaid Program.* Report to the U.S. Senate Subcommittee on Long-Term Care of the Special Committee on Aging, January 5, 1972.
70. U.S. Senate Subcommittee on Long-Term Care of the Special Committee on Aging: *Nursing Home Care in the United States: Failure in Public Policy.* Supporting Paper No. 2, *Drugs in Nursing Homes: Misuse, High Costs, and Kickbacks.* Washington, D.C., U.S. Govt Print Office, 1975.
71. Wertheimer, A. I., Shefter, E., and Cooper, R. M.: The pharmacist as a drug consultant: Three case studies. *Drug Intell Clin Pharm, 7*:58-61, 1973.
72. Wynne, R. D. and Heller, F.: Drug overuse among the elderly: A growing problem. *Perspect Aging, 2*:15-18, 1973.
73. Zimberg, S.: Two types of problem drinkers: Both can be managed. *Geriatrics, 29*:135-137, 1974.

SELECTED BIBLIOGRAPHY

GENERAL

Basen, M. M.: The elderly and drugs—Problem overview and program strategy. *Public Health Rep*, 92:43-48, 1977.

Bourne, P. G.: Drug abuse in the aging. *Perspect Aging*, 2:18-20, 1973.

Butler, R. N.: Public interest report No. 19—The overuse of tranquilizers in older patients. *Int J Aging Hum Dev*, 7:185-187, 1976.

Davis, R. H. and Smith, W. K. (Eds.): *Drugs and the Elderly*. Los Angeles, Ethel Percy Andrus Gerontology Center, U of S Cal, 1973.

Drew, L. R. H.: Alcohol offenders in a Victorian prison. *Med J Aust*, 2:575-578, 1961.

———: Alcoholism as a self-limiting disease. *Q J Stud Alcohol*, 29:956-967, 1968.

Droller, H.: Some aspects of alcoholism in the elderly. *Lancet*, 2:137-139, 1964.

Dupont, R.: Testimony before the Subcommittee on Aging and Subcommittee on Alcoholism and Narcotics of the U.S. Senate Committee on Labor and Public Welfare. Washington, D.C., 1976.

Epstein, L. J., Mills, C., and Simon, A.: Antisocial behavior of the elderly. *Compr Psychiatry*, 11:36-42, 1970.

Gaitz, C. M. and Baer, P. E.: Characteristics of elderly patients with alcoholism. *Arch Gen Psychiatry*, 24:372-378, 1971.

Heller, F. J. and Wynne, R.: Drug misuse by the elderly. In Senay, E., Shorty, V., and Alksne, H. (Eds.): *Developments in the Field of Drug Abuse*. Cambridge, Massachusetts, Schenkman, 1975.

Isbister, J.: Testimony before the Subcommittee on Aging and Subcommittee on Alcoholism and Narcotics of the U.S. Senate Committee on Labor and Public Welfare, Washington, D.C., 1976.

Kayne, R. C.: Drugs and the aged. In Burnside, I. M. (Ed.): *Nursing and the Aged*. New York, McGraw-Hill, 1976.

Lenhart, D. G.: The use of medications in the elderly population. *Nurs Clin North Am*, 11:135-143, 1976.

Mayfield, D. G.: Alcohol problems in the aging patient. In Fann, W. E. and Maddox, G. L. (Eds.): *Drug Issues in Geropsychiatry*. Baltimore, Williams & Wilkins, 1974.

National Institute on Alcohol and Alcoholism: *Alcohol and Health*. Washington, D.C., U.S. Govt Print Office, 1974.

National Institute on Drug Abuse: *Drug Use and the Elderly: Perspectives and Issues*. Proceedings of The Conference on Drug Use and the

Elderly, National Institute on Drug Abuse, Rockville, Maryland, June 12-13, 1975.

Nithman, C. J., Parkhurst, V. E., and Sommes, F. B.: Physicians' prescribing habits: Effects of Medicare. *JAMA, 217*:585-587, 1971.

Pascarelli, E. F.: Alcoholism and drug addiction in the elderly. *Geriatr Focus, 11*:1, 4-5, 1972.

―――: Drug dependence: An age-old problem compounded by old age. *Geriatrics, 29*:109-115, 1974.

Pascarelli, E. F. and Fisher, W.: Drug dependence in the elderly. *Int J Aging Hum Dev, 5*:347-356, 1974.

Petersen, D. M. and Whittington, F. J.: Drug use among the elderly: A review. *J Psychedelic Drugs, 9*:25-37, 1977.

Rosenfelt, R. H., Kastenbaum, R., and Kempler, B.: The untestables: Methodological problems in doing research with the aged. *Gerontologist, 4*:72-74, 1964.

Rosin, A. J. and Glatt, M. M.: Alcohol excess in the elderly. *Q J Stud Alcohol, 32*:53-59, 1971.

Ross, B. and Linn, M. W.: A scale for the measurement of attitudes toward drugs. *Int J Addict, 8*:821-830, 1973.

Ross, B., Greenwald, S. R., and Linn, M. W.: The elderly's perception of the drug scene. *Gerontologist, 13*:368-371, 1973.

Salzman, C., Shader, R. I., Kochansky, G., and Cronin, D. M.: Rating scales for psychotropic drug research with geriatric patients: Mood ratings. *J Am Geriatr Soc, 20*:209-215, 1972.

Seliger, R. V.: Alcoholism in the older age groups. *Geriatrics, 3*:166-170, 1948.

Shropshire, R. W.: The hidden faces of alcoholism. *Geriatrics, 30*:99-102, 1975.

Smith, M. C.: Portrayal of the elderly in prescription drug advertising: A pilot study. *Gerontologist, 16*:329-334, 1976.

Wynne, R. D. and Heller, F.: Drug overuse among the elderly: A growing problem. *Perspect Aging, 2*:15-18, 1973.

Zimberg, S.: The elderly alcoholic. *Gerontologist, 14*:221-224, 1974.

―――: The geriatric alcoholic on a psychiatric couch. *Geriatr Focus, 11*:1, 6-7, 1972.

―――: Two types of problem drinkers: Both can be managed. *Geriatrics, 29*:135-137, 1974.

GERIATRIC PHARMACOLOGY

Aisenberg, R. and Kastenbaum, R.: Value problems in geriatric psychopharmacology. *Gerontologist, 4*:75-77, 1964.

Asnes, D. P.: Psychopharmacology in the aged: Use of major psychotropic medications in treatment of the elderly: Case examples. *J Geriatr Psychiatry, 7*:189-202, 1974.

Bender, A. D.: Geriatric pharmacology: Age and its influence on drug action in adults. *Drug Info Bull*, 3:153-158, 1969.

———: Pharmacologic aspects of aging: A survey of the effects of increasing age on drug activity in the elderly. *J Am Geriatr Soc*, 16:1331-1339, 1968.

———: Pharmacodynamic principles of drug therapy in the aged. *J Am Geriatr Soc*, 22:296-303, 1974.

Berman, P. M. and Kirsner, J. B.: Recognizing and avoiding adverse gastrointestinal effects of drugs. *Geriatrics*, 29:59-62, 1974.

Branson, H. K.: The place of the placebo in geriatric nursing. *Hosp Mgmt*, 98:34-37, 1964.

Bressler, R. and Palmer, J.: Drug interactions in the aged. In Fann, W. E. and Maddox, G. L. (Eds.): *Drug Issues in Geropsychiatry*. Baltimore, Williams & Wilkins, 1974.

Briganti, F. J.: Side effects of drugs used by the elderly. In Davis, R. H. and Smith, W. K. (Eds.): *Drugs and the Elderly*. Los Angeles, Ethel Percy Andrus Gerontology Center, U of S Cal, 1973.

Burch, G.: A review of drug-related neurologic disorders in the elderly. In Fann, W. E. and Maddox, G. L. (Eds.): *Drug Issues in Geropsychiatry*. Baltimore, Williams & Wilkins, 1974.

Busse, E. W.: Hope for rejuvenation. In Fann, W. E. and Maddox, G. L. (Eds.): *Drug Issues in Geropsychiatry*. Baltimore, Williams & Wilkins, 1974.

Chen, K. K.: Principles of pharmacology as applied to the aged. In Stieglitz, E. J. (Ed.): *Geriatric Medicine*. Philadelphia, Saunders, 1943.

Cole, J. O. and Stotsky, B. A.: Improving psychiatric drug therapy: A matter of dosage and choice. *Geriatrics*, 29:74-78, 1974.

Daniel, R.: Psychiatric drug abuse and use in the aged. *Geriatrics*, 25:144-158, 1970.

Davis, J. M.: Psychopharmacology in the aged: Use of psychotropic drugs in geriatric patients. *J Geriatr Psychiatry*, 7:145-149, 1974.

Davison, W.: Drug hazards in the elderly. *Gerontol Clin*, 7:257-264, 1965.

———: Pitfalls to avoid in prescribing drugs for the elderly. *Geriatrics*, 30:157-158, 1975.

DeGraff, A. C.: Drug therapy of cardiovascular disease. *Geriatrics*, 29:51-54, 1974.

Drug metabolism and increasing age. *Br Med J*, 2:581, 1975.

Eisdorfer, C.: Observations on the psychopharmacology of the aged. *J Am Geriatr Soc*, 23:53-57, 1975.

Eisdorfer, C. and Fann, W. E. (Eds.): *Psychopharmacology and Aging*. New York, Plenum Pr, 1973.

Fann, W. E.: Pharmacotherapy in older depressed patients. *J Gerontol*, 31:304-310, 1976.

Fann, W. E. and Lake, C. R.: Drug-induced movement disorders in the elderly: An appraisal of treatment. In Fann, W. E. and Maddox, G. L.

(Eds.): *Drug Issues in Geropsychiatry*. Baltimore, Williams & Wilkins, 1974.
Fann, W. E. and Maddox, G. L. (Eds.): *Drug Issues in Geropsychiatry*. Baltimore, Williams & Wilkins, 1974.
Fann, W. E., Wheless, J. C., and Richman, B. W.: Treating the aged with psychotropic drugs. *Gerontologist*, 16:322-328, 1976.
Freeman, J. T.: *Clinical Principles and Drugs in the Aging*. Springfield, Thomas, 1963.
———: Some principles of medication in geriatrics. *J Am Geriatr Soc*, 22:289-295, 1974.
Friend, D. G.: Drug therapy and the geriatric patient. *Clin Pharmacol Ther*, 2:832-836, 1961.
Gibson, I. and O'Hare, M. N.: Prescription of drugs for old people at home. *Gerontol Clin*, 10:271-280, 1968.
Greenblatt, D. L., Dominick, J. R., Stotsky, B. A., and DiMascio, A.: Phenothiazine-induced dyskinesia in nursing home patients. *J Am Geriatr Soc*, 16:27-34, 1968.
Hall, M.: Use of drugs in elderly patients. *NY J Med*, 75:67-71, 1975.
Hall, M. R. P.: Drug therapy in the elderly. *Br Med J*, 4:582-584, 1973.
———: Drugs in the elderly. *Gerontol Clin*, 16:1-2, 1974.
Hodkinson, H. M.: Biomedical side effects of drugs in the elderly. *Gerontol Clin*, 16:175-178, 1974.
Hollister, L. E.: Drugs for mental disorders in old age. *JAMA*, 234:195-198, 1975.
Holloway, D. A.: Drug problems in the geriatric patient. *Drug Intell Clin Pharm*, 8:632-642, 1974.
Howell, T. H.: Analgesics, hypnotics, and sedatives. *J Gerontol*, 16:395, 1961.
Janowsky, D. M., El-Yousef, K., and Davis, J. M.: Side effects associated with psychotropic drugs. In Fann, W. E. and Maddox, G. L. (Eds.): *Drug Issues in Geropsychiatry*. Baltimore, Williams & Wilkins, 1974.
Kastenbaum, R., Slater, P. E., and Aisenberg, R.: Toward a conceptual model of geriatric psychopharmacology: An experiment with thioridazine and dextro-amphetamine. *Gerontologist*, 4:68-71, 1964.
Lamy, P. P.: Geriatric drug therapy. *Clin Med*, 81:52-57, 1974.
———: *Geriatric Medicine*. Morton Grove, Illinois, Audio Medicus, 1977.
Lamy, P. P. and Kitler, M. E.: Drugs and the geriatric patient. *J Am Geriatr Soc*, 19:23-30, 1971.
Lamy, P. P. and Vestal, R. E.: Drug prescribing for the elderly. *Hosp Prac*, 11:111-118, 1976.
Lasagna, L.: Drug effects as modified by aging. *J Chronic Dis*, 3:567-574, 1956.
Learoyd, B. M.: Psychotropic drugs and the elderly patient. *Med J Aust*, 1:1131-1133, 1972.

Lehmann, H. E.: Psychometric tests in evaluation of brain pathology, response to drugs. *Geriatrics*, 25:142-147, 1970.
Lipshitz, K. and Kline, N. S.: Psychopharmacology in geriatrics. In Clark, W. E. and Del Giudice, V. (Eds.): *Principles of Psychopharmacology.* New York, Academic Pr, 1970.
Means, B. J. and Lamy, P. P.: Ophthalmic drugs for the geriatric patient. *Clin Med*, 82:30-35, 1975.
Modell, W.: Introduction: Use of drugs in the elderly. *Geriatrics*, 29:50, 1974.
Morrant, J. G.: Medicines and mental illness in old age. *Can Psychiatr Assoc J*, 20:309-312, 1975.
Nelson, J. J.: Relieving select symptoms of the elderly. *Geriatrics*, 30:133-142, 1975.
Pfeiffer, E.: Use of drugs which influence behavior in the elderly: Promises, pitfalls, and perspectives. In Davis, R. H. and Smith, W. K. (Eds.): *Drugs and the Elderly.* Los Angeles, Ethel Percy Andrus Gerontology Center, U of S Cal, 1973.
Pratt, R.: Antibiotics in the elderly patient. *Geriatrics*, 12:341-349, 1957.
Raskind, M. and Eisdorfer, C.: Psychopharmacology of the aged. In Simpson, L. L. (Ed.): *Drug Treatment of Mental Disorders.* New York, Raven, 1976.
Ritschel, W. A.: Pharmacokinetic approaches to drug dosing in the aged. *J Am Geriatr Soc*, 24:344-354, 1976.
Robinson, D. B.: Evaluation of certain drugs in geriatric patients: Effects of chlorpromazine, reserpine, pentylenetetrazol U.S.P., and placebo on eighty-four female geriatric patients in a state hospital. *Arch Gen Psychiatry*, 1:41-46, 1959.
Rosen, H. J.: Mental decline in the elderly: Pharmacotherapy (ergot alkaloids versus papaverine). *J Am Geriatr Soc*, 23:169-174, 1975.
Rudd, T. N.: Use of drugs in the older age groups. *Pharmaceutical J*, 132:507-508, 1961.
Salzman, C., Shader, R. I., and Perlman, M.: Psychopharmacology and the elderly. In Shader, R. I. and DiMascio, A. (Eds.): *Psychotropic Drug Side Effects.* Baltimore, Williams & Wilkins, 1970.
Schmidt, C. W.: Psychiatric problems of the aged. *J Am Geriatr Soc*, 22:355-359, 1974.
Schwid, S. A. and Gifford, R. W.: The use and abuse of antihypertensive drugs in the aged. *Geriatrics*, 22:172-182, 1967.
Seager, C. P.: Chlorpromazine in treatment of elderly psychotic women. *Br Med J*, 1:882-885, 1955.
Seneca, H.: Management of infections and infestations in the elderly. *J Am Geriatr Soc*, 18:798-815, 1970.
Slater, P. E., and Kastenbaum, R.: Paradoxical reactions to drugs: Some personality and ethnic correlates. *J Am Geriatr Soc*, 14:1016-1034, 1966.

Stern, F. H.: Sleep-inducing properties of a non-barbiturate analgesic/sedative preparation in elderly patients. *Clin Med*, 79:31-33, 1972.
Stotsky, B.: Use of psychopharmacologic agents for geriatric patients. In DiMascio, A. and Shader, R. I. (Eds.): *Clinical Handbook of Psychopharmacology*. New York, Science House, 1970.
Terri, G. and Franzine, D.: General considerations on drug therapy in the elderly. *J Gerontol*, 20:474-477, 1972.
Triggs, E. J. and Nation, R. L.: Pharmacokinetics in the aged: A review. *J Pharmacokinet Biopharm*, 3:387-418, 1975.
Triggs, E. J., Nation, R. L., Long, A., and Ashley, J. J.: Pharmacokinetics in the elderly. *Eur J Clin Pharmacol*, 8:55-62, 1975.
Wade, O. L.: Drug therapy in the elderly. *Age Aging*, 1:65-73, 1972.
Webb, W. L.: The use of psychopharmacological drugs in the aged. *Geriatrics*, 26:95-103, 1971.
Weg, R.: Drug interactions with the changing physiology of the aged: Practice and potential. In Davis, R. H. and Smith, W. K. (Eds.): *Drugs and the Elderly*. Los Angeles, Ethel Percy Andrus Gerontology Center, U of S Cal, 1973.
Whanger, A. D.: Vitamins and vigor at 65 plus. *Postgrad Med*, 53:167-172, 1973.

EPIDEMIOLOGY

Bahr, H. M. and Caplow, T.: *Old Men Drunk and Sober*. Washington Square, New York, NY U Pr, 1974.
Bahr, H. and Garret, G. R.: *Women Alone: The Disaffiliation of Urban Females*. Lexington, Massachusetts, Lexington Bks, 1976.
Bailey, M. B., Haberman, P. W., and Alksne, H.: The epidemiology of alcoholism in an urban residential area. *Q J Stud Alcohol*, 26:19-40, 1965.
Balter, M. B. and Levine, J.: The nature and extent of psychotropic drug usage in the U.S. *Psychopharmacol Bull*, 5:3-14, 1969.
Bateman, N. I. and Petersen, D. M.: Factors related to outcome of treatment for hospitalized white male and female alcoholics. *J Drug Issues*, 2:66-74, 1972.
─────: Variables related to outcome of treatment for hospitalized alcoholics. *Int J Addict*, 6:215-224, 1971.
Cahalan, D., Cisin, I. H., and Crossley, H. M.: *American Drinking Practices*. New Brunswick, New Jersey, Rutgers Center of Alcohol Studies, 1969.
Cahalan, D. and Room, R.: *Problem Drinking Among American Men*. New Brunswick, New Jersey, Rutgers Center of Alcohol Studies, 1974.
Chambers, C. D.: *An Assessment of Drug Use in the General Population*. New York, New York State Narcotic Addiction Control Commission, 1971.

Chambers, C. D. and Griffey, M.: Use of legal substances within the general population: The sex and age variables. *Addict Dis*, 2:7-19, 1975.

Dunnell, K. and Cartwright, A.: *Medicine Takers, Prescribers and Hoarders.* London, Routledge & Kegan Paul, 1972.

Gorwitz, K., Bahn, A., Warthen, F. J., and Cooper, M.: Some epidemiological data on alcoholism in Maryland. *Q J Stud Alcohol*, 31:423-443, 1970.

Guttman, D.: *A Survey of Drug Taking Behavior of the Elderly.* Washington, D.C., Catholic U, 1977.

Hindmarch, I.: Drugs and their abuse. Age groups particularly at risk. *Br J Addict*, 67:209-214, 1962.

Johnson, L. A. and Goodrich, C. H.: Use of alcohol by persons 65 years and over, upper east side of Manhattan. Cited by National Institute on Alcohol Abuse and Alcoholism: *Alcohol and Health.* Washington, D.C., U.S. Govt Print Office, 1974.

Knupfer, G. and Room, R.: Age, sex, and social class as factors in amount of drinking in a metropolitan community. *Soc Prob*, 12:224-240, 1964.

Locke, B. Z., Kramer, M., and Pasamanick, B.: Alcoholic psychoses among first admissions to public mental hospitals in Ohio. *Q J Stud Alcohol*, 21:457-474, 1960.

Malzberg, B.: A study of first admissions with alcoholic psychoses in New York State, 1943-1944. *Q J Stud Alcohol*, 8:274-295, 1947.

McCusker, J., Cherubin, C. E., and Zimberg, S.: Prevalence of alcoholism in general municipal hospital population. *NY J Med*, 71:751-754, 1971.

Mellinger, G. D., Balter, M. B., Parry, H. J., Manheimer, D. I., and Cisin, I. H.: An overview of psychotherapeutic drug use in the United States. In Josephson, E. and Carroll, E. E. (Eds.): *Drug Use: Epidemiological and Sociological Approaches.* Washington, D.C., Hemisphere Pub, 1974.

Parry, H. J.: Use of psychotropic drugs by United States adults. *Public Health Rep*, 83:799-810, 1968.

Petersen, D. M. and Thomas, C. W.: Acute drug reactions among the elderly. *J Gerontol*, 30:552-556, 1975.

Schuckit, M. A.: Geriatric alcoholism and drug abuse. *Gerontologist*, 17:168-174, 1977.

Schuckit, M. A. and Miller, P. L.: Alcoholism in elderly men: A survey of a general medical ward. *Ann NY Acad Sci*, 273:558-571, 1975.

Selzer, M. L. and Holloway, W. H.: A follow-up of alcoholics committed to a state hospital. *Q J Stud Alcohol*, 18:98-120, 1957.

Siassi, I., Crocetti, G., and Spiro, H. R.: Drinking patterns in a blue collar population. *Q J Stud Alcohol*, 34:917-926, 1973.

Simon, A., Epstein, L. J., and Reynolds, L.: Alcoholism among the geriatric mentally ill. *Geriatrics*, 23:125-131, 1968.

Task Force on Prescription Drugs: *The Drug Users.* Washington, D.C., U.S. Govt Print Office, 1968.

———: The Drug Users and the Drug Prescribers. Washington, D.C., U.S. Govt Print Office, 1971.

Warheit, G. J., Arey, S. A., and Swanson, E.: Patterns of drug use: An epidemiologic overview. *J Drug Issues,* 6:223-237, 1976.

Whittier, J. R. and Korenyi, C.: Selected characteristics of aged patients: A study of mental hospital admissions. *Compr Psychiatry,* 2:113-120, 1961.

Wolff, S. and Holland, L.: A questionnaire follow-up of alcoholic patients. *Q J Stud Alcohol,* 25:108-118, 1964.

Zax, M., Gardner, E. A., and Hart, W. T.: Public intoxication in Rochester: A survey of individuals charged during 1961. *Q J Stud Alcohol,* 25: 669-678, 1964.

SELF-MEDICATION AND COMPLIANCE

Brand, F. N., Smith, R. T., and Brand, P. A.: Effect of economic barriers to medical care on patients' non-compliance. *Public Health Rep,* 92:72-78, 1977.

Curtis, E. B.: Medication errors made by patients. *Nurs Outlook,* 9:290-291, 1961.

Davis, M. S.: Physiologic, psychological, and demographic factors in patient compliance with doctor's orders. *Med Care,* 6:115-122, 1968.

———: Variations in patients' compliance with doctors' orders: Analysis of congruence between survey responses and results of empirical investigations. *J Med Educ,* 41:1037-1048, 1966.

———: Variations in patients' compliance with doctors' advice: An empirical analysis of patterns of communication. *Am J Public Health,* 58:274-288, 1968.

Davidson, J. R.: Presentation and packaging of drugs for the elderly. *J Hosp Pharmacol,* 31:180-184, 1973.

———: Trial of self-medication in the elderly. *Nurs Times,* 11:391-392, 1974.

Hemminki, E. and Heikkila, J.: Elderly people's compliance with prescriptions, and quality of medication. *Scand J Soc Med,* 3:87-92, 1975.

Kelly, P.: An experiment in self-medication for older people. *Can Nurse,* 68:41-43, 1972.

Latiolais, C. J. and Berry, C. C.: Misuse of prescription medications by outpatients. *Drug Intell Clin Pharm,* 3:270-277, 1969.

Lofholm, P.: Self-medication by the elderly. In Davis, R. H. and Smith, W. K. (Eds.): *Drugs and the Elderly.* Los Angeles, Ethel Percy Andrus Gerontology Center, U of S Cal, 1973.

Neely, E. and Patrick, M. L.: Problems of aged persons taking medications at home. *Nurs Res,* 17:52-55, 1968.

Schwartz, D.: The elderly patient and his medications. *Geriatrics,* 20:517-520, 1965.

Schwartz, D., Wang, M., Zeitz, L., and Goss, M. E. W.: Medication errors made by elderly chronically ill patients. *Am J Public Health*, 52:2018-2029, 1962.

Stewart, R. B. and Cluff, L. E.: A review of medication errors and compliance in ambulant patients. *Clin Pharmacol Ther*, 13:463-468, 1967.

Thumin, F. and Wims, E.: The perception of the common cold, and other ailments and discomforts, as related to age. *Int J Aging Hum Dev*, 6:43-50, 1975.

DRUG MANAGEMENT AND EDUCATION

Anderson, W. F.: Administration, labeling and general principles of drug prescription in the elderly. *Gerontol Clin*, 16:4-9, 1974.

Brimigion, J.: The role of the nurse in long-term drug management. In Fann, W. E. and Maddox, G. L. (Eds.): *Drug Issues in Geropsychiatry*. Baltimore, Williams & Wilkins, 1974.

Carruth, B., Williams, E. P., Mysak, P., and Boudreaux, L.: *Community Care Providers and the Older Problem Drinker*. Paper presented to The General Sessions of the Alcohol and Drug Problems Association of North America, September 23-28, 1973.

Compton, B.: The role of the family nurse practitioner in the drug management of the elderly patient in a rural community. In Fann, W. E. and Maddox, G. L. (Eds.): *Drug Issues in Geropsychiatry*. Baltimore, Williams & Wilkins, 1974.

Forbes, J. A.: Prescribing for the elderly in general practice and the problems of record keeping. *Gerontol Clin*, 16:14-17, 1974.

Gaeta, M. J. and Gaetano, R. J.: *The Elderly, Their Health and the Drugs in Their Life*. Dubuque, Iowa, Kendall-Hunt, 1977.

Jessup, L. E.: Nursing responsibilities in drug administration. In Davis, R. H. and Smith, W. K. (Eds.): *Drugs and the Elderly*. Los Angeles, Ethel Percy Andrus Gerontology Center, U of S Cal, 1973.

Kabat, H. F.: Nursing's role in geriatric drug therapy. *Geriatr Nurs*, 3:8-11, 1967.

Maultsby, M. C.: Decreasing prescription suicides or a behavioral approach to irrational fears and insomnia. *J Am Med Wom Assoc*, 27:416-419, 1972.

Miller, M. B.: Clinical observations on drug management of psychiatrically ill aged patients. In Fann, W. E. and Maddox, G. L. (Eds.): *Drug Issues in Geropsychiatry*. Baltimore, Williams & Wilkins, 1974.

Plant, J.: Educating the elderly in safe medication use. *Hospitals*, 51:97-102, 1977.

Plutchik, R., McCarthy, M., Hall, B. H., and Silverberg, S.: Evaluation of a comprehensive psychiatric and health care program for elderly welfare tenants in a single-room occupancy hotel. *J Am Geriatr Soc*, 21:452-459, 1973.

Subby, P.: *A Community Based Program for the Chemically Dependent Elderly.* Paper presented to The North American Congress on Alcohol and Drug Problems, San Francisco, December, 1975.

Zimberg, S.: The psychiatrist and medical home care: Geriatric psychiatry in the Harlem ghetto. *Am J Psychiatry, 127*:1062-1066, 1971.

———: Outpatient geriatric psychiatry in the urban ghetto with nonprofessional workers. *Am J Psychiatry, 125*:1697-1702, 1969.

NURSING HOMES

Apfeldorf, M. and Hunley, P. J.: Application of MMPI alcoholism scales to older alcoholics and problem drinkers. *J Stud Alcohol, 36*:645-653, 1975.

Apfeldorf, M., Hunley, P., and Cooper, G. D.: Disciplinary problems in a home for older veterans: Some psychological aspects in relation to drinking behavior. *Gerontologist, 12*:143-147, 1972.

Archambaut, G. F.: The law concerning dangerous drugs in nursing homes. *Hosp Mgmt, 101*:68-81, 1966.

Barton, R. and Hurst, L.: Unnecessary use of tranquilizers in elderly patients. *Br J Psychiatry, 112*:989-990, 1966.

Chien, C. P., Jung, K., and McMahon, N.: *Psychiatric Drug Practice in Nursing Homes: Rational and Irrational.* Paper presented to the annual meeting of the American Geriatrics Society, San Francisco, 1977.

Harrington, L. G. and Price, A. C.: Alcoholism in a geriatric setting. I. Disciplinary problems, marital status and income level. *J Am Geriatr Soc, 10*:197-200, 1962.

———: Alcoholism in a geriatric setting. II. Education, military service and employment records. *J Am Geriatr Soc, 10*:201-203, 1962.

———: Alcoholism in a geriatric setting. III. Age on admission to domiciliary, length of stay, diagnosis, and sources of income. *J Am Geriatr Soc, 10*:204-206, 1962.

———: Alcoholism in a geriatric setting. IV. Incidence of drug addiction and disease. *J Am Geriatr Soc, 10*:207-208, 1962.

———: Alcoholism in a geriatric setting. V. Incidence of mental disorders. *J Am Geriatr Soc, 10*:209-211, 1962.

Kabat, H. F., Kidder, S. W., Martilla, J. K., and Stewart, J. E.: *Drug Utilization Review in Skilled Nursing Facilities: A Manual System for Performing Sample Studies of Drug Utilization.* Washington, D.C., U.S. Department of Health, Education and Welfare, 1975.

Kayne, R. C. and Cheung, A.: An application of clinical pharmacy in extended care facilities. In Davis, R. H. and Smith, W. K. (Eds.): *Drugs and the Elderly.* Los Angeles, Ethel Percy Andrus Gerontology Center, U of S Cal, 1973.

Kent, E. A. and Gitman, L.: Chemopsychiatric institutional care of the aged. *Geriatrics, 15*:480-486, 1960.

Linn, M., Linn, B. S., and Greenwald, S. R.: The alcoholic patient in the nursing home. *Aging Hum Dev, 3*:273-278, 1972.

Lucas, M.: Alcoholism in homes for the aged in the Paris region. *Rev Alcoholisme, 14*:268-284, 1969.

Milliren, J. W.: Some contingencies affecting the utilization of tranquilizers in long-term care of the elderly. *J Health Soc Behav, 18*:206-211, 1977.

Moss, B. B.: Effective drug administration as viewed by a physician/administrator. In Davis, R. H. and Smith, W. K. (Eds.): *Drug and the Elderly.* Los Angeles, Ethel Percy Andrus Gerontology Center, U of S Cal, 1973.

Moss, F. E. and Halamandaris, V. J.: Nursing home drugs: Pharmaceutical Russian roulette. In Moss, F. E. and Halamandaris, V. J.: *Too Old, Too Sick, Too Bad.* Germantown, Maryland, Aspen Systems, 1977.

Townsend, C.: *Old Age: The Last Segregation.* New York, Grossman, 1971.

Twigg, W. C.: Alcoholism in a home for the aged. *Geriatrics, 14*:391-395, 1959.

U.S. Senate Subcommittee on Long-Term Care of the Special Committee on Aging: *Nursing Home Care in the United States: Failure in Public Policy.* Supporting Paper No. 2: *Drugs in Nursing Homes: Misuse, High Costs, and Kickbacks.* Washington, D.C., U.S. Govt Print Office, 1975.

Whanger, A. D.: Drug management of the elderly in state hospitals. In Fann, W. E. and Maddox, G. L. (Eds.): *Drug Issues in Geropsychiatry.* Baltimore, Williams & Wilkins, 1974.

ALCOHOL THERAPY

Becker, P. W. and Cesar, J. A.: Use of beer in geriatric psychiatric patient groups. *Psychol Rep, 33*:182, 1973.

Beer and the geriatric patient. *Geriatr Nurs, 4*:14-18, 1968.

Black, A. L.: Altering behavior of geriatric patients with beer. *Northwest Med, 68*:453-456, 1969.

Burrill, R. H., McCourt, J. F., and Cutter, H. S. G.: Beer: A social facilitator for PMI patients? *Gerontologist, 14*:430-431, 1974.

Chien, C. P.: Beer more effective than drugs as psychologic prop to elderly. *Geriatr Focus, 9*:5-6, 1970.

———: Psychiatric treatment for geriatric patients: "Pub" or drug? *Am J Psychiatry, 127*:1070-1075, 1971.

Chien, C. P., Stotsky, B. A., and Cole, J. O.: Psychiatric treatment for nursing home patients: Drug, alcohol, and milieu. *Am J Psychiatry,' 130*:543-548, 1973.

Kastenbaum, R.: Beer, wine, and mutual gratification in the gerontopolis. In Kent, D. P., Kastenbaum, R., and Sherwood, S. (Eds.): *Research, Planning and Action for the Elderly.* New York, Behavioral Pub, 1972.

———: Wine and fellowship in aging: An exploratory action program. *J Hum Relations, 13*:266-276, 1965.

Kastenbaum, R. and Slater, P. E.: Effects of wine on the interpersonal behavior of geriatric patients: An exploratory study. In Kastenbaum, R. (Ed.): *New Thoughts on Old Age*. New York, Springer Pub, 1964.

Mishara, B. L. and Kastenbaum, R.: Wine in the treatment of long-term geriatric patients in mental institutions. *J Am Geriatr Soc, 22*:88-94, 1974.

Mishara, B. L., Kastenbaum, R., Baker, F., and Patterson, R. D.: Alcohol effects in old age: An experimental investigation. *Soc Sci Med, 9*:535-547, 1975.

Leake, C. D. and Silverman, M.: The clinical use of wine in geriatrics. *Geriatr Focus, 6*:175-180, 1967.

Volpe, A. and Kastenbaum, R.: Beer and TLC. *Am J Nurs, 67*:100-103, 1967.

ILLEGAL DRUGS

Ball, J. C., Bates, W. M., and O'Donnell, J. A.: Characteristics of hospitalized narcotic addicts. *HEW Indicators*:17-26, 1966.

Ball, J. C. and Lau, M. P.: The Chinese narcotic addict in the United States. *Soc Forces, 45*:68-72, 1966.

Bean, P.: The drug takers 1920-1970. In Bean, P.: *The Social Control of Drugs*. New York, Wiley, 1974.

Capel, W. C. and Stewart, G. T.: The management of drug abuse in aging populations: New Orleans findings. *J Drug Issues, 1*:114-121, 1971.

Capel, W. C., Goldsmith, B. M., Wadell, K. J., and Stewart, G. T.: The aging narcotic addict: An increasing problem for the next decades. *J Gerontol, 27*:102-106, 1972.

Glick, M. A.: Elderly addicts are treatable. *J Addict Res Found Ontario, 3*:8, 1974.

O'Donnell, J. A.: *Narcotic Addicts in Kentucky*. Washington, D.C., Public Health Service Publ No. 1881, U.S. Govt Print Office, 1969.

Pescor, M. J.: Physician drug addicts. *Dis Nerv Syst, 3*:173-174, 1942.

Snow, M.: Maturing out of narcotic addiction in New York City. *Int J Addict, 8*:921-938, 1973.

Winick, C.: Physician narcotic addicts. *Soc Problems, 9*:174-186, 1961.

———: Maturing out of addiction. *Bull Narc, 14*:1-7, 1962.

———: The life cycle of the narcotic addict and of addiction. *Bull Narc, 16*:1-11, 1964.

SUICIDE

Bean, P.: Accidental and intentional self-poisoning in the over sixty age group. *Gerontol Clin, 15*:259-267, 1973.

Benson, R. A. and Brodie, D. C.: Suicide by overdoses of medicines among the aged. *J Am Geriatr Soc,* 23:304-308, 1975.

Matthew, H.: Poisoning in the home by medicaments. *Br Med J,* 2:788-790, 1966.

Maultsby, M. C.: Decreasing prescription suicides or a behavioral approach to irrational fears and insomnia. *J Am Med Wom Assoc,* 27:416-419, 1972.

Patterson, R. D., Abrahams, R., and Baker, F.: Preventing self-destructive behavior. *Geriatrics,* 29:115-121, 1974.

NAME INDEX

Addis, G. J., 64, 76
Agulnik, P. L., 62, 71
Aisenberg, R., 16, 20, 26
Alexander, W. D., 70, 71
Alksne, H., 26, 29, 30, 38
Alling, E., 70, 72
Altemeier, W. A., 85, 92
Anderson, H., 156, 158, 161
Apogi, E., 54, 71
Atchley, R. C., 41, 50
Avant, G. R., 60, 75
Ayd, F. J., 58, 71

Bahn, A., 28, 30, 39
Bailey, M. B., 29, 30, 38
Baker, A. B., 57, 76
Ball, J. C., 16, 21, 22, 26
Ball, W. L., 115, 124
Ballingal, D. L. K., 64, 76
Balter, M. B., 194, 218
Baragar, F. D., 68, 71
Barcus, F. E., 193, 216
Barney, J. L., 211, 216
Baron, J. H., 53, 71
Barrett, R. E., 57, 79
Barsky, A. J., 115, 124
Bartlett, E., 181, 189
Barton, R., 14, 16, 20, 26, 41, 50, 149, 150
Basen, M. M., 24, 26
Bateman, N. I., 25, 26
Bauer, G. E., 63, 65, 71
Bauer, R. B., 57, 77
Bechgaard, P., 63, 71
Beck, K. D., 64, 76
Becker, P. W., 30, 36, 38, 202, 216
Beers, R. F., 68, 77
Belcher, J. C., 94, 103
Bell, W. G., 214, 216
Bender, A. D., 53, 54, 55, 71

Benson, R. A., 181, 189
Bernstein, A., 191, 192, 193, 196, 204, 205, 206, 216, 218
Bernstein, J. M., 68, 76
Berry, C. C., 97, 103, 119, 125
Berry, K., 59, 74
Bilck, M. K., 57, 76
Birren, J. E., 72
Bland, J., 54, 72
Blum, R. H., 192, 216
Blumberg, J. E., 156, 158, 161
Blume, S. B., 38
Bogdonoff, M., 8
Bondareef, W., 54, 72
Boudreaux, L., 32, 34, 38
Bourg, C. J., 181, 189
Bourne, P. G., 24, 26, 141, 150, 196, 216
Brady, E. S., 164, 176, 183, 189
Brand, F. N., 198, 214, 216
Brand, P. A., 198, 214, 216
Breme, J. T., 60, 72
Brenner, J., 168, 176
Brest, A. N., 54, 74
Briant, R. H., 65, 72
Brickner, P. W., 151, 161
Bridge, T. P., 207, 217
Brod, J., 62, 72
Brodie, B. B., 53, 54, 74, 78
Brodie, D. C., 181, 189
Brody, E. M., 200, 216
Brody, H., 54, 72
Brody, S. J., 208, 210, 216, 217
Browdy, S., 210, 217
Brown, M. I., 159, 161
Brown, W. T., 61, 72
Bruce, R., 70, 72
Buffaloe, W. J., 59, 75
Burack, R., 204, 205, 212, 217
Burnside, I. M., 152, 161, 176
Busse, E. W., 206, 217
Butler, R. N., 156, 159, 161

Cahalan, D., 18, 26, 28, 30, 38
Caird, F. I., 66, 72, 78
Callahan, J. A., 67, 77
Canada, A. T., 107, 125
Candy, S., 198, 218
Cantor, M. H., 182, 189
Capel, W. C., 14, 16, 23, 24, 26, 41, 50, 154, 161
Caranasos, G. J., 56, 68, 72
Carlson, J. R., 195, 217
Carroll, E. E., 219
Carruth, B., 32, 34, 38
Carter, M., 70, 72
Catalano, P., 108, 119, 120, 125
Cesar, J. A., 30, 36, 38, 202, 216
Chambers, C. D., 16, 18, 21, 26, 42, 50, 207, 217
Chen, K. K., 96, 103
Cherubin, C. E., 31, 32, 39
Chesrow, E. J., 60, 72
Cheung, A., 199, 208, 209, 213, 217, 218
Chien, C., 30, 37, 39
Chinn, A., 161
Cisin, I. H., 18, 26, 28, 30, 38, 194, 218
Citrenbaum, M., 155, 161
Clesceri, L., 68, 77
Close, C., 101, 102, 103
Cluff, L. E., 56, 68, 70, 72, 77, 90, 93, 98, 104
Cohen, C. I., 181, 182, 184, 189
Cole, E., 185, 189
Cole, J. O., 30, 37, 39, 58, 77
Compton, W. A., 105, 124
Connor, P. K., 64, 76
Conway, J., 56, 63, 64, 72
Cooke, A. R., 68, 69, 72, 73
Cooper, M., 28, 30, 39
Cooper, R. M., 206, 213, 220
Corbin, K. B., 68, 74
Crane, G. E., 58, 72
Crawley, H. K., III, 199, 217
Crocetti, G., 29, 31, 39
Cromie, B. W., 60, 73
Crossley, H. M., 18, 26, 28, 30, 38
Currie, G., 96, 103
Curtis, E. B., 119, 124

Curwen, M. P., 60, 73
Cutler, R. W., 57, 73

Danian, M., 101, 102, 103
Daniel, R., 20, 26, 58, 59, 62, 72
Davidson, S., 66, 72
Davis, J. M., 58, 61, 72, 75, 181, 189
Davis, M. S., 121, 124, 198, 217
Davis, R. H., 20, 26, 41, 50, 141, 144, 150, 176, 189, 218, 219
Davison, C., 68, 70, 72, 73
Dawborn, J. K., 64, 73
Debus, G., 60, 75
De Graff, A. C., 54, 66, 73
de Groot, M. H. L., 61, 73
de Lint, J., 28, 33, 39
Dennis, E., 64, 76
Denzin, N. K., 213, 217
de Ropp, R. S., 193, 217
de Tocqueville, A., 192, 217
Deutschberger, S., 94, 103
Devas, M. B., 95, 103
de Vries, H. A., 183, 189
Dimascio, A., 58, 62, 71, 73
Di Palma, J. R., 73
Dittert, L. W., 86, 92
Dixon, A. St. J., 68, 69, 78
Dixon, W. M., 120, 124
Dollery, C. T., 65, 72
Doluisio, J. T., 86, 92
Donegan, T. J., 108, 124
Douglas, J. D., 204, 205, 207, 208, 212, 217
Dowling, H. F., 205, 217
Doyle, A. E., 64, 73
Drapkin, A., 114, 124
Drew, L. R. H., 28, 39
Dreyfus, E. G., 119, 120, 125
Drizmal, H., 70, 78
Droller, H., 35, 39
Drummond, E. E., 156, 158, 161
Duckham, J. M., 107, 124
Duke University Center for the Study of Aging and Human Development, 6, 7
DuPont, R., 167, 176
Duthie, J. R., 68, 71

Name Index

Duvoisin, R. C., 57, 79
Dymock, I. W., 64, 76

Ebringer, A., 64, 73
Eckel, F. M., 199, 217
Efron, D. H., 75
Eimerl, T. S., 9, 12
Eisdorfer, C., 6, 12, 72, 77, 155, 161, 217
Eisenmenger, W. J., 114, 124
Elizan, T. S., 57, 76
Ellinwood, E. H., 207, 217
El-Yousef, M. K., 58, 61, 72
Ensminger, B., 169, 177
Epstein, L., 7, 12
Epstein, L. J., 29, 30, 31, 39, 204, 205, 206, 218
Ewy, G. A., 66, 73
Exton-Smith, A. N., 60, 73

Fahn, S., 57, 73
Fann, W. E., 5, 6, 12, 20, 26, 41, 50, 58, 61, 72, 77, 141, 150, 217
Faris, D., 33, 39
Fields, W. S., 75
Finkle, B. S., 59, 73
Fischer, W., 17, 23, 27, 141, 150
Flack, H. L., 119, 120, 125
Foner, A., 41, 50
Ford, R. V., 63, 76
Forner, D., 55, 73
Forrest, F. M., 59, 73
Forrest, I. S., 59, 73
Fostiropolous, G., 68, 76
Fox, F. J., 204, 205, 212, 217
Francke, D. E., 213, 217
Freeman, J. T., 96, 103
Friedman, S. A., 54, 73
Friend, D. G., 55, 63, 67, 68, 69, 73
Frimpter, G. W., 114, 124
Fulda, T. R., 204, 217
Fulop, M., 114, 124

Gaitz, C. M., 76
Galloway, D. B., 59, 64, 79
Garai, P. R., 205, 217

Garland, J., 10, 12
Garvin, J. S., 57, 75
Georgia Office of Aging, 95, 103
Gerber, M., 67, 73
Gibson, I., 55, 73
Gifford, R. W., 56, 62, 63, 64, 65, 78
Gillis, M., 151, 162
Gillum, R. F., 115, 124
Gilman, A., 79
Glaser, B. G., 153, 162
Glatt, M. M., 34, 35, 36, 39
Goldberg, A., 10, 13
Goldsmith, B. M., 14, 16, 23, 26, 41, 50, 154, 161
Goldstein, R. C., 68, 69, 79
Goldstein, S. W., 89, 93
Goodman, L., 9, 12
Goodman, L. S., 79
Goran, S., 57, 73
Gorrod, J. W., 164, 176
Gorwitz, K., 28, 30, 39
Goss, M. E. W., 97, 103, 164, 166, 177
Goulston, K., 69, 73
Graham, J. H., 193, 217
Granerus, A., 57, 73
Granville-Grossman, K. L., 58, 70, 73
Graupner, K. I., 59, 77
Green, L. W., 171, 176
Greenberger, M., 169, 177
Greenblatt, D. J., 58, 73
Greenblatt, S., 165, 176, 214, 217
Greenwald, S. R., 37, 39, 178, 189
Greer, H. D., 68, 74
Greiner, A. C., 59, 74
Griener, G. E., 119, 124
Griner, P. F., 118, 125
Gusfield, J. R., 190, 218

Haberman, P. W., 29, 30, 38
Haider, I., 61, 74
Halamandaris, V. J., 199, 200, 201, 202, 219
Hall, M. R. P., 53, 74, 96, 103
Hallberg, J. C., 173, 176
Halpern, M. M., 64, 74
Hamilton, L. D., 54, 58, 59, 74
Hamm, B., 166, 176

Hansson, L., 64, 74
Hapgood, D., 202, 219
Harris, R., 208, 218
Harrison, T. S., 64, 74
Hastings, G., 99, 103
Healy, K. M., 171, 176
Hecht, A., 167, 176
Heider, C. H., 54, 63, 74, 76
Heimsoth, V., 64, 76
Heller, F. J., 19, 24, 26, 27, 141, 150, 154, 162, 206, 213, 220
Herrmann, G. R., 66, 67, 74
Herxheimer, A., 77, 78
Hillery, G. A., Jr., 179, 189
Himwich, H. E., 54, 74
Hobby, G. L., 86, 92
Hodes, B., 108, 124
Hodkinson, H. M., 60, 73
Hodkinson, M., 157, 162
Hoehn, M. M., 57, 79
Hogben, C. A. M., 53, 54, 74, 78
Hofner, P. E., 105, 115, 125
Hollenhorst, R. W., 67, 77
Hollister, L. E., 59, 74
Holman, R. B., 64, 74
Hoobler, S. W., 64, 74
Hornykiewicz, O., 57, 74
Hoyumpa, A., 60, 75
Hunyor, S. N., 64, 74
Hurst, L., 14, 16, 20, 26, 41, 50, 149, 150
Hurwitz, N., 55, 66, 74
Hussar, D. A., 98, 99, 100, 103, 115, 124
Huxley, A., 192, 218

Ilahi, M. M., 57, 75
Isbister, J., 166, 176
Ishak, K. G., 69, 78
Jacobson, E., 55, 74
Janke, W., 60, 75
Jankowski, S. M., 193, 216
Janowsky, D. S., 58, 61, 72
Jarcho, L. W., 59, 78
Jeffers, A., 59, 64, 79
Jick, H., 60, 75
Johnson, A. N., 212, 218

Johnson, A. W., 59, 75
Johnson, N., 108, 124
Johnston, C. I., 64, 73
Jorgensen, L. A., 212, 218
Joseph, C., 57, 75
Josephson, E., 219
Julius, S., 64, 74

Kabat, H. F., 210, 218
Kane, R. L., 212, 218
Kantor, D. L., 108, 124
Kapadia, G. G., 66, 73
Kaplitz, S. E., 60, 72
Kastenbaum, R., 16, 20, 26, 198, 218
Katz, L. N., 67, 75
Kayne, R. C., 164, 176, 199, 218
Keenan, R. E., 57, 75
Kennedy, R. D., 66, 78
Kent, D. P., 203, 218
Keyes, J. W., 55, 64, 75
Kidder, S. W., 210, 218
Kim, K. E., 64, 76
Kinard, S. A., 64, 76
Kitler, M. E., 20, 26
Klawans, H. L., 57, 75
Klein, D. F., 61, 75
Klerman, G. L., 194, 218
Kline, N. S., 58, 75
Klotz, U., 60, 75
Koller, M. R., 41, 50
Kopp, H., 63, 71
Kosek, J. C., 59, 74
Kosman, M. E., 64, 65, 75
Kramer, M., 28, 30, 39
Kurland, L. T., 56, 57, 75
Kuwahara, J., 212, 218

Lader, M., 58, 78
Lader, S., 58, 78
Lamy, P. P., 20, 26
Langrell, H. M., 57, 75
La Piana, J. C., 86, 92
Lasagna, L. C., 115, 118, 124, 125, 164, 176
Latiolais, C. J., 97, 103, 119, 125
Lau, M. P., 16, 22, 26

Name Index

Lawson, A. A. H., 68, 75
Leake, C. D., 99, 103
Learoyd, B. M., 16, 20, 26, 56, 62, 76
Lee, H. A., 107, 124
Lehmann, H. E., 55, 76
Lennard, H. L., 7, 12, 191, 192, 193, 196, 204, 205, 206, 216, 218
Lesshafft, C. T., 107, 125
Levine, J., 58, 77
Levine, R. R., 68, 76
Lewis, M. I., 156, 159, 161
Lewis, S. M., 68, 69, 78
Libsch, L. R., 57, 73
Linkewich, J. A., 119, 120, 125
Linn, B. S., 37, 39
Linn, M. W., 37, 39, 178, 189
Lisansky, E. T., 38, 39
Locke, B. Z., 28, 30, 39
Loewenson, R. B., 57, 76
Lucarotti, R. L., 105, 115, 125
Lullin, M., 66, 73
Lumpaneli, A. E., 114, 124

MacArthur, J. G., 64, 76
MacDougall, A. I., 64, 76
Mackay, N., 64, 76
MacLean, N., 68, 75
MacLennan, W. J., 64, 76
MacNeill, R. M., 96, 103
Maddox, G. L., 5, 6, 12, 20, 26, 41, 50, 141, 150, 190
Malahy, B., 97, 103
Malzberg, B., 28, 30, 39
Mandel, G., 68, 73
Manheimer, D. I., 194, 218
Mann, K., 66, 77
Manso, C., 69, 76
Marcus, F. I., 66, 73
Marsh, W. W., 67, 71, 76
Martilla, J. K., 210, 218
Martin, W. E., 57, 76
Mashford, M. L., 64, 73
Master, A., 67, 76
Maultsby, M. C., 208, 218
Mazzullo, J. M., 118, 125
McCusker, J., 31, 32, 39
McGlothlin, W. H., 194, 218

McHale, M. K., 107, 125
McLeod, D. C., 199, 217
Mechanic, D., 207, 213, 218
Mehl, C., 42, 50
Mellinger, G. D., 194, 218
Melmon, K. L., 80, 92
Mendelson, M. A., 200, 201, 202, 219
Merquet, P., 64, 76
Mettlin, C. J., 213, 217
Metzger, A. L., 68, 69, 79
Meyler, L., 77, 78
Miller, E. M., 57, 58, 76
Miller, P. L., 31, 32, 39
Milliren, J. W., 14, 17, 20, 26
Millis, J., 133, 138
Mills, C., 29, 30, 39
Mintz, M., 167, 176
Mitchell, A. D., 54, 76
Modell, W., 11, 12
Moller, D. N., 119, 120, 125
Monathe, V. V., 119, 125
Mones, R. J., 57, 76
Moore, P., 62, 71
Moreland Act Commission, 126, 138
Moss, F. E., 199, 200, 201, 202, 219
Moulding, T., 121, 125
Moyer, J. H., 63, 64, 76
Mudie, E. W., 96, 103
Muller, C., 205, 209, 210, 213, 219
Murphree, O. D., 59, 77
Musci, J., 60, 72
Musser, R. D., 164, 177
Mydrick, J., 69, 76
Myers, E. N., 68, 76
Mysak, P., 32, 34, 38

Naaman, 197
National Institute on Alcohol Abuse and Alcoholism, 28, 39
Neelsen, J., 63, 71
New York State Legislature, 126, 138
Newman, S. C., 42, 50
Nieburg, H. A., 57, 76

O'Donnell, J. A., 17, 21, 27
O'Neill, J. J., 164, 177
Onek, J., 169, 177

Onesti, G., 64, 76
Osler, W., 192, 219

Palmers, H., 63, 64, 72
Palmore, E., 198, 219
Parry, H. J., 194, 218
Parsons, T., 197, 219
Pasamanick, B., 28, 30, 39
Pascarelli, E. F., 17, 23, 27, 141, 150
Paul, B. N., 70, 77
Payne, B. P., 187, 189
Peck, C., 119, 125
Peele, R., 59, 77
Percy, C. H., 195, 208, 209, 219
Perlman, L. V., 67, 71, 76
Pescor, M. J., 17, 22, 27
Petersen, D. M., 14, 17, 19, 25, 26, 27, 42, 50, 207, 217
Petrie, J. C., 59, 64, 79
Pevey, K., 63, 76
Pfeiffer, E., 141, 144, 150, 195, 200, 219
Pharmaceutical Manufacturers Association, 204, 219
Plant, J., 208, 219
Plotz, P. H., 69, 78
Porter, I. H., 68, 69, 78
Prange, A. J., 61, 77
Prescott, L. F., 68, 77
Prien, R. F., 58, 77, 214, 219
Prisco, H. M., 105, 115, 125
Proudfoot, A. T., 56, 77

Quick, A. J., 68, 77
Quinney, R., 204, 219

Rabin, D. L., 97, 103
Raizner, A. E., 54, 73
Ransom, D. C., 204, 205, 206, 218
Reid, J. L., 65, 72
Rensberger, B., 6, 13
Resch, J. A., 57, 76
Reveno, W. S., 57, 77
Reynolds, L., 29, 31, 39

Reynolds, R. C., 70, 77
Richardson, H. L., 59, 77
Richardson, M. E., 59, 77
Riley, M. W., 41, 50
Roback, G. A., 167, 177
Robertson, D. M., 67, 77
Rodstein, M., 198, 219
Rosen, H., 54, 73
Rosenbaum, H., 57, 77
Rosenberg, B., 119, 125
Rosenberg, J. M., 66, 77
Rosenthal, M., 7, 12
Rosin, A. J., 34, 35, 36, 39
Rosow, I., 180, 182, 189
Ross, B., 178, 189
Russell, A. S., 69, 77
Ryder, C. F., 216, 219

Sabatini, R., 60, 72
Salter, W. T., 54, 77
Samter, M., 68, 77
Sannerstedt, R., 56, 63, 72
Schanker, L. S., 53, 54, 74, 78
Schear, M. J., 57, 79
Scheiner, J., 85, 92
Schmidt, R. F., 60, 78
Schmidt, W., 28, 39
Schmidt, W. R., 59, 78
Schneker, S., 60, 75
Schuckit, M. A., 24, 27, 31, 32, 39
Schwab, M., 164, 165, 177
Schwartz, D., 55, 56, 78, 97, 103, 164, 166, 177
Schwid, S. A., 56, 62, 63, 64, 65, 78
Scott, J. T., 68, 69, 78
Seaman, W. E., 69, 78
Seidenberg, R., 206, 219
Seidl, L. G., 90, 93
Senay, E., 26
Sergeant, H. G. S., 58, 70, 73
Shader, R. I., 58, 73
Shefter, E., 206, 213, 220
Sheiner, L. B., 119, 125
Shenker, D., 57, 75
Shepherd, M., 58, 78
Shepherd's Center, The, 185, 189
Sherwood, S., 218

Name Index

Shillito, E., 64, 74
Shore, H., 214, 219
Shore, P. A., 53, 78
Shorty, V., 26
Shoup, L. K., 105, 115, 125
Siassi, I., 29, 31, 39
Siegel, G. J., 57, 76
Silverman, C., 60, 78
Simon, A., 29, 30, 31, 33, 39
Slater, P. E., 16, 20, 26
Smith, D. E., 42, 50
Smith, G., 70, 71
Smith, J. W., 90, 93
Smith, M. A., 69, 77
Smith, M. C., 206, 220
Smith, P. K., 70, 72
Smith, R. T., 198, 214, 216
Smith, W. K., 20, 26, 41, 50, 141, 144, 150, 176, 189, 218, 219
Solomon, H. M., 89, 93
Solomon, N. A., 54, 73
Spiro, H. R., 29, 31, 39
Stanaszek, W. F., 95, 101, 103
Stannard, C., 200, 201, 220
Stewart, G. T., 14, 16, 23, 24, 26, 41, 50, 154, 161
Stewart, J. E., 210, 218
Stewart, R. B., 56, 68, 72, 98, 104
Stieglitz, E. J., 103
Storm van Leeuwen, W., 70, 78
Stotsky, B. A., 30, 37, 39
Straus, R., 38, 40
Strauss, A. L., 153, 162
Stredling, P., 120, 124
Sturge, R. A., 69, 77
Subby, P., 208, 220
Sun, D. C. H., 64, 68, 78
Surawicz, B., 66, 72
Svanborg, A., 57, 73
Sy, W., 54, 73

Talalay, P., 12, 217
Taranta, A., 69, 76
Tarpie, A. G. G., 64, 76
Task Force on the Pharmacist's Clinical Role, 100, 104

Task Force on Prescription Drugs, 15, 18, 27, 41, 47, 50, 164, 177
Taylor, B. B., 66, 78
Termini, B., 181, 189
Teteberg, B., 212, 218
Thomas, C. W., 14, 17, 19, 27
Thomas, J. H., 66, 78
Thorson, J., 161
Tibbitts, C., 41, 50
Tice, L. F., 111, 125
Tocco, D. J., 53, 54, 74
Townsend, C., 20, 27, 196, 199, 200, 201, 220

U.S. Department of Health, Education, and Welfare, 9, 13
U.S. General Accounting Office, 199, 220
U.S. Senate Special Committee on Aging, 6, 7, 11, 13
U.S. Senate Subcommittee on Long-Term Care, 126, 127, 138, 199, 200, 206, 207, 211, 220

Van Der Velde, C. D., 62, 78
Vedder, C. B., 41, 50
Velk, W. L., 54, 76
Vernon, S., 54, 78
Verzar, F., 55, 73
Vidt, D. G., 62, 63, 65, 78
Vogel, M. E., 60, 78
Vogt, M., 64, 74
von Loetzen, I. S., 59, 77

Waddell, K. J., 14, 16, 23, 26, 41, 50, 154, 161
Wade, O. L., 55, 66, 74
Wake, C. D., 167, 177
Wagner, J. G., 84, 93
Waldie, P., 10, 13
Walker, T. G., 96, 103
Wallin, D. G., 119, 120, 125
Walters, P. G., 107, 125
Wang, M., 97, 103, 164, 166, 177

Ward, H. P., 68, 74
Warren, R., 179, 189
Warthen, F. J., 28, 30, 39
Webb, W. L., 55, 59, 60, 61, 78
Webster, J., 59, 64, 79
Weiss, J., 108, 125
Wenzel, D., 96, 97, 104
Wertheimer, A. I., 206, 213, 220
Whiting, B., 10, 13, 64, 76
Wilkinson, G. R., 60, 75, 86, 92
Williams, E. P., 32, 34, 38
Williams, G. R., 56, 79
Williams, R. T., 53, 79
Wilson, C. H., 69, 79
Wilson, J. T., 116, 125
Winick, C., 14, 17, 21, 22, 27
Wise, W., 67, 75
Wolfe, J. D., 68, 69, 79

Wood, P. N. H., 69, 79
Wood, R., 117, 125
Woodbury, D. M., 70, 79
Wotten, I. D. P., 120, 124
Wright, N., 56, 77
Wynne, R. D., 19, 24, 26, 27, 141, 150, 154, 162, 206, 213, 220

Yahr, M. D., 57, 79
Yao, L., 66, 73

Zeitz, L., 97, 103, 164, 166, 177
Zimberg, S., 31, 32, 34, 35, 36, 39, 40, 203, 220
Zimmerman, H. J., 68, 69, 79
Zimmerman, M., 60, 78

SUBJECT INDEX

Absorption of drugs, 53-54, 58, 82, 83-85, 96, 119, 164
Acetominophen, 144
Acetylcholine, 90
Acetylsalicylic acid, 68-70, 97, 107, 144, 147
Acute drug reactions
   age patterns of incidence, 19, 42-45, 49, 55, 80
   age patterns of risk, 55, 80
   alcohol—other drugs, 43, 45, 49
   and drug interactions, 81, 114
   hospital emergency admissions for, 41-50
   incidence of, 9, 10, 17, 19, 41-50, 98, 99, 128, 154
   lack of research on, 47-48
   number of substances involved, 43-45, 49, 56, 164
   and physiological changes, 99, 128, 164
   prevention of, 10, 101, 113, 155, 156
   primary drug related to, 45-47, 49
   race patterns of incidence, 42-44, 49
   resulting from self-administration, 153
   sex patterns of incidence, 42-44, 48, 49
   and suicide attempt, 43, 45, 47, 49
   unreported and untreated, 19, 48, 56
Adsorption of drugs, 83, 85, 89
Adult day care
   prevention of drug misuse, 187
Adult education
   prevention of drug misuse, 187-188
Adverse drug reactions (*see* Acute drug reactions)
Age
   and alcohol misuse, 28
   and alcohol use, 15, 28
   and incidence of acute drug reactions, 19, 42-45, 49, 55, 80
   and incidence of alcoholism, 28, 30
   lack of pharmacological information related to, 11-12, 212
   and medication errors, 98
   and prevalence of alcoholism, 29-33
   and risk of acute drug reaction, 55, 80
   and use of non-prescription drugs, 15, 47
   and use of prescription drugs, 15, 47, 97
Aged (*see* Elderly)
Aging
   normal process of, 96, 141-142, 164, 165, 195-196
   process of and drug interactions, 80, 128
   process of and drug misuse, 20, 164, 165
   process of and pharmacological efficacy, 41, 53-55, 58, 96
   stresses of, 34, 35, 36, 38, 95, 141-142, 164, 165, 180-182
Agitation, 144, 146-147, 148
Agonist drug, 89, 90
Alcohol, 5, 7, 14, 15, 19, 23, 25, 28-40, 43, 45, 49, 69, 91, 145, 153, 154, 180, 181, 183, 192, 202, 203
   acute reactions with other drugs, 43, 45, 49
   age pattern of misuse, 28
   age pattern of use, 15, 28
   consumption rate related to alcoholism, 33
   epidemiology of use, 28-33
   recreational use of, 7
   review of research on the elderly, 28-38

sociability effects of, 30, 36-38, 153, 202-203
Alcohol abuse
  factors related to, 35
  research interest in, 5
Alcohol therapy (see Alcohol, sociability effects of)
Alcoholics
  death rates of, 28
Alcoholism
  and accidents, 28
  age incidence of, 28, 30
  age prevalence of, 29-33
  and cardiovascular disorders, 28
  and cirrhosis of the liver, 28
  and consumption rate of alcohol, 33
  early-onset type (see Elderly alcoholics, early-onset type)
  iatrogenic, 37, 38, 203
  late-onset type (see Elderly alcoholics, late-onset type)
  and pneumonia, 28
  prevention of, 36-38
  and psychiatric hospitalization, 29, 30, 31
  rate among older women, 29, 34
  spontaneous remission of (see Alcoholism, as a self-limiting disease)
  and suicide, 28
  treatment of, 35-36, 37, 38
Alka-Seltzer, 160
Alternatives to institutionalization, 214
Aluminum hydroxide gel, 83
AMA (American Medical Association), 209
American society
  overmedication of, 192-195
Amitriptyline, 60, 144
Ammonium chloride, 90
Amphetamines, 18, 89, 90, 113, 143, 193
Analgesics, 18, 19, 46, 47, 50, 67-70, 88, 91, 120, 127, 143, 144, 147, 196, 203
Anectine, 90
Antacids, 83, 84, 96
Antagonist drug, 89, 90

Antianxiety drugs, 59-60
Antibiotics, 83, 84, 122
Anticholinergics (see Antispasmodics)
Anticoagulants, 81, 86, 88
Antidepressants, 18, 30, 35, 38, 60-61, 143, 144, 146, 209 (see also Tricyclic antidepressants)
Antidiabetic drugs, 88, 89, 134
Antidiarrheals, 83
Antihistamines, 88, 122, 143, 144
Antihypertensive drugs, 62-65, 89, 134
Antimanic drugs, 61-62
Antiobesity drugs, 116
Anti-Parkinson drugs, 56-58
Antipsychotic drugs, 58-59
Antispasmodics, 81, 89, 122
Anturane, 87
Anxiety, 144, 148, 161
Arthritis, 152
Aspirin (see Acetylsalicylic acid)
Atabrine, 87
Atropine, 46, 90
Attitude towards drugs
  and belief in physician infallibility, 193
  desire for panacea solutions, 192-194
  factors related to, 193-195
  and mass media, 194-195
  and medication errors, 55
  need for skepticism, 208
Aventyl, 60, 144

Banthine, 90
Barbiturates, 18, 19, 23, 91, 113, 143, 181, 193, 205
Beer
  used to promote sociability, 30, 36-38, 202-203
Belladonna, 97, 122
Bendroflumethiazide, 63
Benzedrine, 18
Benzodiazepines, 59-60, 143
Bereavement
  and drinking problems, 34
Biotransformation of drugs (see Metabolism of drugs)
Bishydroxycoumarin, 88, 89

Subject Index

Bureau of Narcotics and Dangerous Drugs (*see* Drug Abuse Warning Network)
Butaperazine, 58
Butazolidin, 86, 87

Caffeine, 143, 170
Cancer, 152
Cardiac glycosides, 66-67, 91, 122
Cardiovascular disorders, 28, 57, 61, 64, 65, 66, 67, 70, 144, 152
Cardiovascular drugs, 15, 62-67, 134
Catapres, 64
Cathartics, 97
Cerebrovascular disease, 152
Chemical straight-jacket, 127, 130
"Chemophilia," 193
Chemopsychiatric era, 193
Chloral hydrate, 144
Chlordiazepoxide, 18, 59, 144
Chlorothiazide, 63
Chlorpheniramine, 122
Chlorpromazine, 20, 58-59, 122, 144
Chlorthalidone, 63
Cholestyramine, 84
Cirrhosis, 28
Clark's Rule, 164
Clonidine, 64, 65
CNS-acting drugs (*see* Psychoactive drugs)
Cocaine, 18, 46
Codeine, 18
Community, 178-180
Community health programs, 31, 32, 35, 36, 160, 186, 188, 208, 213-214
Community mental health center, 25, 28, 31, 32, 34
Compazine, 58
Complexation of drugs, 83, 84, 85
Compliance, 105, 115-116, 119-123, 135, 145, 169, 198, 199, 214
  factors related to, 67, 71, 116, 119-123, 198
Confusion, 58, 61, 68, 144, 146, 156
Conspiracy theory, 204

Containers for drugs, 117-118, 134, 165, 212
Coumadin, 87
Coumarin, 86

Dalmane, 144
Darvon, 18, 19, 46, 47, 50
DAWN (*see* Drug Abuse Warning Network)
Day care (*see* Adult day care)
Deanol, 58
Declomycin, 83, 85
Decongestants, 170
Delirious reactions (*see* Confusion)
Demeclocycline hydrochloride, 83, 85
Demerol, 22, 46
Depressants, 55, 91
Depression, 6, 38, 57, 58, 60, 61, 64, 65, 144, 145-146, 147, 148, 156, 161, 209, 211
  and drinking problems, 34, 35, 145
  and drug problems, 145, 156
  and medication errors, 55
  and number of drugs prescribed, 48
  and suicide, 146, 181
Desipramine, 60, 144
Detail men (*see* Drug detail men)
Detoxication (*see* Detoxification of drugs)
Detoxification of drugs, 96, 155-156
Dexamyl, 18
Dexedrine, 18, 20, 46
Dextroamphetamine, 16
Diazepam, 18, 46, 59, 60, 144
Dicloxacillin, 84, 86
Dicumarol, 88
Diet pills, 18
Digitalis, 66, 90, 91, 97, 99, 122
Digoxin, 66, 122
Dilaudid, 23
Diphenhydramine, 122
Distribution of drugs, 58, 82, 85-87, 164
Diuretics, 18, 63-65, 91, 122, 134
Diuril, 63
Dopamine, 57
Dopar, 56

Doriden, 18
Doxepin, 30, 37, 60, 144
Drug abuse
  lack of research on the elderly, 14, 24-25, 41, 141
  research interest in, 5
  social influences on, 180-182
Drug Abuse Warning Network (DAWN), 19, 208
Drug addiction
  "maturing out" of, 14, 21-22, 23
Drug advertising, 194-195, 205-207
  directed at nursing home administrators, 206-207
  directed at physicians, 197, 205, 206, 213
  Federal Trade Commission control of, 108, 205, 212-213
  negative portrayal of elderly, 206
  susceptibility of the elderly, 206, 215
Drug attitudes (see Attitude toward drugs)
Drug awareness center for the elderly, 175
Drug containers
  as drug control devices, 134, 212
  problems with, 117-118, 165, 212
Drug detail men, 197, 205, 209
Drug disc, the, 10
Drug-drug interactions (see Drug interactions)
Drug education
  in an academic setting, 172-173
  curriculum development, 169-171
  of the elderly, 120, 121, 163-176, 182, 208
  of health professionals, 8, 9-10, 130, 149, 183, 195, 208-209, 211
  instructor selection, 173
  practical considerations in, 172-175
Drug efficacy
  variables related to, 9, 41, 54-55, 96, 212
Drug industry
  advertising by, 108, 194-195, 197, 205-207, 212-213, 215
  development of new drugs, 204-205, 212

and drug policy, 191, 203-207
  need for research in geriatric pharmacology, 212
  number of psychoactives produced, 193
  profit motive of, 204-207
  questionable marketing tactics of, 204-207
  relationship to physicians, 197, 205, 206, 213
  tendency to medicalize human behavior, 206
Drug information network, 209
Drug interactions, 20, 41, 64, 80-92, 99-100, 101-102, 114, 137, 209
  by accelerated metabolism, 87-88
  and acute drug reactions, 81, 114
  and the aging process, 80, 128
  alcohol-other drugs, 19, 43, 45, 69
  definition of, 81
  during absorption, 83-85
  during distribution, 85-87
  during excretion, 90-91
  during transport (see Drug interactions, during distribution)
  effects of, 86, 87, 88, 89, 156
  with foods, 156
  incidence of, 128
  increased evidence of, 82
  by inhibited metabolism, 88-89
  and multiple diseases, 80-81
  and multiple drug therapy, 81
  other types, 91
  potentiating effects, 20
  prescription with nonprescription drugs, 101-102
  prevention of, 10, 101
  at the receptor site, 89-90
  risk of, 80, 196
  strategy for minimizing, 91-92
  warning system for, 10
Drug management, 8-9, 10, 11, 20, 25, 41, 212
Drug metabolism
  age patterns, 20, 53-54, 58, 60, 82, 87-89, 164
Drug misuse
  and the aging process, 20, 164, 165

Subject Index

by the elderly, 5, 12, 190, 195
correlates of, 215
incidence and prevalence, 24-25
lack of standard definition, 15
and mystification, 206
need for research, 214-215
in nursing homes (*see* Nursing homes)
of the elderly, 6, 12, 190, 195
programs to prevent, 183-188
research interest in, 5
and social disorganization, 194
Drug monitoring system, 208, 210, 211
Drug overdose (*see* Acute drug reactions)
Drug policy, 190-216
and the drug industry, 191, 203-207
and nursing homes, 191, 198-203
and physicians, 191, 195-198
proposals, 208-215
Drug reactions (*see* Acute drug reactions)
Drug-related disorders (*see* Iatrogenic illness, resulting from drug therapy)
Drugs
absorption of, 53-54, 58, 82, 83-85, 96, 119, 164
acute reactions to (*see* Acute drug reactions)
administration errors in nursing homes, 6, 127, 199, 211
adsorption of, 83, 85, 89
conditions treatable with, 144-148
controlled substances, 113
cost of, 10-11, 15, 41, 97, 100, 109-110, 116, 121-123, 170, 210, 211, 212, 213
detoxification of, 96, 155-156
distribution of, 58, 82, 85-87, 164
efficacy of, 9, 41, 54-55, 96, 212
excretion of, 53-54, 58, 60, 82, 83, 90-91, 96, 164
generic-trade name controversy, 122-123, 170, 171
illegal (*see* Illegal drugs)
instructions for use, 56, 113, 118-119, 135-136, 159-160

labeling (*see* Drugs, instructions for use)
legal (*see* Legal drugs)
metabolism of, 20, 53-54, 58, 60, 82, 87-89, 164
in nursing homes (*see* Nursing homes)
outdated, 114-115
pain management with, 144, 147, 158-159, 203
placebo effect, 9, 97, 215
recreational use of, 7, 178
review of research on the elderly, 14-25
self-administration (*see* Self-administration of drugs)
self-medication (*see* Self-medication)
side effects of, 6, 20, 41, 53-71, 81, 99, 112, 114, 120, 143, 144, 155, 156, 164, 165, 196, 209
social message of, 153, 157-158
therapy for terminal illness, 203
unavailability of, 116-117
which influence behavior, 142-145
Drug therapy
geriatric, 96-97
iatrogenic illness from, 7, 37, 41, 56, 96, 98, 141, 195
intent of physicians' prescription, 9
of mental disorders, 41, 142-148
with multiple drugs, 96, 143, 145, 154, 198
proper dosage in the elderly, 164-165, 212
risk-to-benefit ratio, 165
in terminal illness, 203
Drug use
community responsibility for, 178-189
cultural basis of, 191-195
incidence, prevalence, and extent of use, 18, 24-25, 56
lack of research on the elderly, 14, 24, 25, 41
lack of standard definition, 15
in nursing homes (*see* Nursing homes)
societal attitude towards, 166

Drug utilization review system, 209, 210
Drunkenness
  arrests of elderly for, 29-30
Dynapen, 84

Edecrine, 87
Education about drugs (*see* Drug education)
Elavil, 18, 60, 144
Elderly
  causes of death among, 152
  chronic conditions in, 147-151, 214
  drug needs of, 94, 95, 96-97
  drugs most frequently used, 16, 18
  health needs of, 94, 95, 165
  health status of, 94
  home remedies, use of, 215
  institutionalization of, 5, 151, 155, 198-199, 214
  number in community, 163
  problems related to number of drugs prescribed, 48
  reduced drug dosage for, 54, 164-165, 212
  self-diagnosis, 197
  types of drug problems, 97-100
  women (*see* Older women)
Elderly alcoholics
  community agencies, seen in, 29-30
  in a community mental health center, 31, 32
  early-onset type, 34-35
  in a geriatric psychiatry outpatient program, 31, 32
  hospitalization of, 29, 30, 31
  late-onset type, 34-35
  of long-standing (*see* Elderly alcoholics, early-onset type)
  treatment of, 35-36, 37, 38
  types of, 33-35
Elderly drug abusers
  low profile in the community, 25
Elderly narcotic addicts
  low profile in the community, 16, 23, 25
  projected growth in numbers, 23-24

Elimination of drugs (*see* Excretion of drugs)
Epinephrine, 99
Equanil, 144
Esidrix, 91
Eskalith, 61
Ethacrynic acid, 87
Ethchlorvynol, 144
Ethical drugs, 213
Ethyl alcohol (*see* Alcohol)
Excretion of drugs, 53-54, 58, 60, 82, 83, 90-91, 96, 164
Extended care facilities (*see* Nursing homes)

FDA (*see* Food and Drug Administration)
Federal Trade Commission
  control of drug advertising, 108, 205, 212-213
Ferrous sulfate, 83
Flaxedil, 90
Fluphenazine, 144
Flurazepam, 144
Folk medicine, 215
Food and Drug Administration
  control of nonprescription drugs, 108
  regulation of new drugs, 204, 212
  review of nonprescription drugs, 107, 111
Fordham's College at Sixty, 187-188
FTC (*see* Federal Trade Commission)
Furosemide, 91

Gallamine, 90
Gastrointestinal problems, 61, 63, 64, 68, 120, 165
General Accounting Office
  and drug fraud in nursing homes, 202
Generic-trade name controversy, 122-123, 170, 171
Gentamycin, 90
Geriatric drug therapy, 96-97
  proper dosage, 164-165, 212
  risk-to-benefit ratio, 165

Subject Index

Geriatric medicine
  lack of incentive for physicians, 196
  need for medical specialty, 208-209
  number of specialists, 167, 195
  practice of, 95, 195-198
Geriatric nursing
  goals in treatment and medication, 153-154
  nurses' dislike of, 151
  rewards of, 151
Geriatric pharmacology
  need for research by drug industry, 212
Geriatric pharmacy, 128-131
Glue (*see* Inhalants
Glutethemide, 18
Guanethidine, 63, 65, 90

Haldol, 144
Hallucinogens, 18, 46, 49
Haloperidol, 143, 144
Health education, 168-169
Health Maintenance Organizations
  and quality and cost of health care, 210
Hearing impairment, 60, 68
Heart disease (*see* Cardiovascular disease)
Help seeking, 24, 25
Heparin, 83
Heroin, 18, 23, 46, 49
High blood pressure (*see* Hypertension)
HMO (*see* Health Maintenance Organizations)
Home health care (*see* Community health programs)
Hopelessness
  and drinking problems, 35
Hospitals, 16, 17, 19, 20, 21, 22, 23, 25, 28, 29, 30, 31, 32, 34 36-37, 55, 56, 98, 149, 152, 153, 154, 155, 171, 208
  emergency rooms in, 17, 19, 41-50, 82, 106, 165, 171, 208
Hydralazine, 63
Hydrochlorothiazide, 63, 122

HydroDIURIL, 63, 91
Hygroton, 63
Hypertension, 15, 62, 63, 64, 65, 81, 156, 160
Hypnotics, 144, 181
Hypochondriasis, 148
Hypotension, 57, 58, 59, 63, 64, 70, 99, 144

Iatrogenic alcoholism, 37, 38, 203
Iatrogenic illness
  resulting from drug therapy, 7, 37, 41, 56, 96, 98, 141, 195
Ibuprofin, 116
Illegal drugs
  use of, 17, 20-24, 46, 49
Illicit drugs (*see* Illegal drugs)
Illness
  and drinking problems, 34, 36
  drug-induced (*see* Iatrogenic illness)
  multiple among the elderly, 6, 20, 25, 95, 96, 155, 164, 195, 196
  physicians' confusion with aging process, 195-196
Imipramine, 60, 65, 90, 144
Inderal, 90
Indocin, 165
Indomethacin, 135
Inhalants, 46
Institutionalization, 5, 151, 155, 198-199, 214
Intermediate care facilities
  drug distribution system, 134-136
  pharmaceutical services in, 132-136
  resident self-administration of medication in, 132-133
Isabella Geriatric Center
  intermediate care facility, 129, 132-136
  nursing home, 129, 136-138
  pharmaceutical services in, 128-138
  residential facility, 129, 131-132
Ismelin, 65, 90
Isolation (*see* Social isolation)
Isoproterenol, 90
Isuprel, 90

Jackson Memorial Hospital
admissions for acute drug reactions,
41-50

Kaolin pectin mixture, 83
Kaopectate, 83, 84

Labeling of drugs (*see* Drugs,
instructions for use)
Larodopa, 56
Lasix, 91
Laxatives, 107, 122, 154
L-dopa, 56-58, 156
Legal drugs
misuse of, 15, 17, 18-20, 24, 25,
45-49
use of, 15-18, 24-25, 164
Librium, 18, 46, 47, 59, 60, 144
Licit drugs (*see* Legal drugs)
Lincocin, 83, 84
Lincomycin, 83, 84
Lithane, 61
Lithium carbonate, 61, 62, 143, 144
Lithonate, 61
Loneliness
related to drinking problems, 34, 36
Long-term care institutions (*see*
Nursing homes)
Low blood pressure (*see* Hypotension)
LSD, 18, 46
L-3, 4-dihydroxyphenylalanine, 56
L-tryptophan, 57
Luminal, 18, 19

MAO inhibitors, 143
Marijuana, 18
Marital stress
related to drinking problems, 34, 36
Mass media
portrayal of drugs, 194-195
"Maturing out" of addiction, 14, 21-22,
23
Medicaid, 126, 130, 136, 210
coverage of drug costs, 100, 116, 211,
212, 213

and drug fraud in nursing homes,
202
Medicare, 126, 130, 136, 210
coverage of drug costs, 100, 116, 211,
212
and drug fraud in nursing homes, 202
Medication duplication, 98-99, 154-155
Medication errors
by elderly patients, 55, 67, 71, 97-
98, 113, 164
by nurses, 9, 127
by physicians, 6, 9
relationship to age, 98
types of, 55, 98, 127
Mellaril, 18, 20, 58, 144, 200
Mental disorders, 6, 15, 18, 36, 57, 58,
60, 61, 64, 65, 68, 142, 144, 145-
148, 156
assessment of, 148-149
drug treatment of, 41, 142-148
neglect by physicians, 149
Meperidine, 17, 22
Meprobamate, 143, 144
Mescaline, 18
Metabolism of drugs, 20, 53-54, 58, 60,
82, 87-89, 164
Methadone, 16, 17, 23, 46
Methadone maintenance programs
elderly patients in, 17, 23
Methaqualone, 144, 207
Methedrine, 18
Methenamine, 90
Methotrexate, 87
Methyldopa, 63
Methylphenidate, 90, 143, 144
Methyprylon, 144
Milk of magnesia, 122, 154
Miltown, 144
Morphine, 17, 18, 22
Motrin, 116

Narcotic addicts
Chinese-American, 16, 22
elderly, 16, 20-24, 25, 154
middle-aged, 23
physicians, 17, 22
Narcotics, 17, 18, 20-24, 46, 113, 154

Subject Index

Naturetin, 63
Navane, 144
Nicotine, 60, 170
Nighttime activities
   prevention of drug misuse, 184-185
Nitrofurantoins, 90
Noctec, 144
Nocturnal neurosis, 181, 184
Noludar, 144
Nonbarbiturate sedative-hypnotics (see Sedative-hypnotics)
Nonprescription drugs
   age pattern of use, 15, 47
   cost of, 109-110
   factors affecting choice of, 107-110
   Food and Drug Administration control of, 108
   Food and Drug Administration review of, 107, 111
   interactions with prescription drugs, 101-102
   pharmacist advice on, 100, 110, 207
   resulting in acute drug reactions, 45-47
   self-medication with, 105-115, 131, 145, 215
Norepinephrine, 65
Norisodrine, 90
Norpramine, 60, 144
Nortriptyline, 60, 144
Nurses
   determination of patients' drug habits, 154-155
   dislike of geriatric service, 151
   goals in geriatric treatment and medication, 153-154
   medication errors by, 9, 127
   need for geriatric drug education, 9-10, 149, 211
   need for geriatric training, 211
   need for patient medication history, 154-155
   pharmacological training of, 9-10, 130, 149, 211
   responsibility for drug administration, 151-161, 211
   responsibility for prevention of acute drug reactions, 156
   rewards of geriatric service, 151
   role in alleviation of pain, 158-159
   role in overmedication, 156, 201
   role in self-administration of drugs, 159-160
   use of alternatives to drug therapy, 156-157
Nursing homes
   alcohol therapy to promote sociability, 30, 36-38, 202-203
   drug administration errors in, 6, 127, 199, 211
   drug distribution systems in, 127, 136-138, 149, 211
   drug experimentation in, 199
   drug fraud investigated by the General Accounting Office, 202
   drug kickbacks paid by, 128, 201-202, 211
   drug misuse in, 6-7, 19-20, 126-138, 149, 199-203
   and drug policy, 191, 198-203
   drugs most frequently prescribed in, 127
   elderly demand for drugs in, 200
   humanistic approach to patient care, 128, 211
   inadequate control of drugs in, 127-128, 211
   need for enforcement of drug regulations, 210
   need for staff drug education, 149, 211
   ombudsman role in, 211-212
   overmedication of residents, 11, 19-20, 62, 127, 149, 156, 199, 200-201, 214-215
   pharmaceutical services in, 100, 136-138, 201-202, 210-211
   pharmacist's role in, 11, 100, 126-138, 201-202, 210
   prognostic system of cost reimbursement, 212
   public concern with, 126-127, 211-212
   pursuit of profits by, 201-202, 212
   social therapies in, 211, 215
   staff attitudes towards patients, 215

treatment of elderly alcoholics in, 36
undermedication of residents, 198, 199, 214
use of tranquilizers in, 200, 206-207
Nursing home administrators
role in overmedication, 201
targets of drug advertising, 206-207
Nutrition
prevention of drug misuse, 184

Older women, 20, 58-59, 62
and acute drug reactions, 48, 49
alcoholism rate among, 29, 34
and psychoactive drugs, 25
"Old's Rule," 212
Ombudsman
role in nursing homes, 211-212
Opiates, 16, 17, 20, 21
Opium, 18, 22
Opthalmic ointment, 117
Organic brain syndromes, 147-148, 156
Orinase, 87, 88
Overmedication
of American society, 192-195
hypothesis, 194-195
in nursing homes, 11, 19-20, 62, 127, 149, 156, 199, 200-201, 214-215
Over-the-counter drugs (*see* Nonprescription drugs)
Oxazepam, 59
Oxyphenylbutazone, 87

Pain
drug management of, 144, 147, 154, 158-159, 203
Pamaquin, 87
Panwarfin, 87
Paranoid reactions, 144, 146, 147
Parkinson's disease, 56-58, 156
Patient profile card, 101, 131, 134, 137-138
Penicillin, 84, 192
Pentazocine, 144
Percodan, 196
Perphenazine, 58
Pertofrane, 60, 144

Pharmaceutical manufacturers (*see* Drug industry)
Pharmaceutical services, 94-102, 128-131
to intermediate care facility residents, 132-136
to nursing home residents, 100, 136-138, 201-202, 210-211
to residential facility dwellers, 131-132
Pharmacists
as advisors on nonprescription drugs, 100, 110, 207
and drug kickbacks, 128, 201-202, 211
monitoring drug use, 99, 100-102, 207, 213
need for geriatric drug education, 149, 183
and prevention of drug misuse, 213
relationship to nursing homes, 11, 100, 126-138, 201-202, 210
services to community residents, 100-102, 207, 213
Pharmacological Calvinism, 194
Pharmacological efficacy
effect of aging process on, 41, 53-55, 58, 96
role of Food and Drug Administration, 212
Pharmacology
lack of age-related information about, 11-12, 212
training of nurses in, 9-10, 130, 149, 211
training of physicians in, 8, 9-10, 195, 208-209
Phenobarbital, 18, 46, 50, 55, 88, 122
Phenothiazines, 58-59, 143
Phenylbutazone, 86, 87
Physical exercise
prevention of drug misuse, 183-184
Physicians
belief in infallibility of, 193
confusion of disease and aging process, 195-196
and drug policy, 191, 195-198
expectations of, 197

Subject Index

geriatric training of, 195, 208-209
and health education and counseling, 209
in HMOs, 210
inappropriate prescription practices of, 6, 38, 141, 156, 167, 215
lack of incentives to specialize in geriatrics, 196
medication errors by, 9
narcotic addicts, 17, 22
need for geriatric drug education, 149, 183, 195, 208-209
negative attitudes toward elderly, 167-168, 195-196
neglect of mental disorders, 149
and overmedication, 201
patient compliance with drug orders of, 115-116, 198
pharmacological training of, 8, 9-10, 195, 208-209
prescribing patterns, 5-12, 141, 209-210, 214
and psychoactive drugs, 141-150
reliance on drug company information, 197, 213
susceptibility to drug company advertising, 197, 205, 206, 213
tendency to medicalize all aspects of life, 196
therapeutic intent of drug prescriptions, 9
unavailability of, 105-106
unwillingness to diagnose alcoholism, 38
Physician shopping, 197
Pilocarpine, 89, 90
Placebo, 9, 97, 215
Placidyl, 18, 144
Poison Prevention Packaging Act, 117
Potassium, 63, 64, 91
Potassium chloride, 64
Preludin, 18
Prescription drugs
age pattern of use, 15, 47, 97
categories most frequently prescribed, 15, 41
conditions for which prescribed, 15
cost of, 15, 116

errors made by physicians, 6, 9
improperly obtained, 111-112
interactions with nonprescription drugs, 101-102
most commonly prescribed, 18
number psychoactives prescribed, 193
resulting in acute drug reactions, 45-47
Prevention
of acute drug reactions, 10, 101, 113, 155, 156
of alcoholism, 36-38
of drug interactions, 10, 101
of drug misuse, 183-188, 213
"Prn" medication, 158
Pro-Banthine, 90
Prochlorperazine, 58
Prolixin, 144
Propranolol, 90
Protriptyline, 60
Psilocybin, 18
Psychiatric disorders (*see* Mental disorders)
Psychoactive drugs, 16, 18, 19, 24, 25, 30, 37, 46, 47, 49, 56-62, 129, 134, 167, 181, 192, 193, 196, 204
Psychotherapeutic drugs, 192, 194
Psychotogens (*see* Hallucinogens)
Psychotropic drugs (*see* Psychoactive drugs)

Quaalude, 144
Questran, 84
Quinacrine, 87
Quinine, 46

Recreational drugs, 7, 178
Repoise, 58
Reserpine, 64
Residential facilities
pharmaceutical services in, 131-132
Retirement
and drinking problems, 34, 36
Ritalin, 144

Salicylates, 67-70, 86, 87

Secobarbitol, 46, 181
Seconal, 18, 46
Sedative-hypnotics, 16, 18, 37, 88
Sedatives, 19, 46, 47, 49, 113, 127, 143, 146, 200, 207
Self-administration of drugs, 105, 115-124, 154, 163
  in intermediate care facilities, 132-133
  nurses' role in, 159-160
  problems of, 153, 165
  resulting in acute drug reactions, 153
Self-medication, 94, 97, 98, 105-124, 163-164, 166
  advantages of, 110-111
  problems with, 20, 106-107, 165, 166
  reasons for, 105-106
  with nonprescription drugs, 105-115, 131, 145, 215
  without medical supervision, 111-115
Serax, 59
Serpasil, 64
Shepherd's Center, the
  model for volunteer services, 185-187
Sick role, 152, 153, 197
Sinequan, 60, 144
Skilled nursing facility (see Nursing home)
Sleep disturbance, 144, 145, 147, 148
Social death, 153
Social isolation
  and drinking problems, 35
Social policy (see Drug policy)
Sodium amobarbital, 46
Sodium bicarbonate, 90
Soma, 192
Sopor, 144
Stelazine, 58, 144
Steroids, 134
Stimulants, 16, 18, 20, 46, 55, 143, 144
Streptomycin, 83
Stresses of aging
  and late-onset alcoholism, 34, 35, 36, 38
Substance abuse (see Drug abuse)
Succinylcholine, 90
Suicide
  and alcoholism, 28
  and depression, 146, 181
  and the use of hypnotics, 144, 181
  incidence of, 146, 180
Suicide attempts
  factors related to, 181
  resulting in acute drug reactions, 43, 45, 47, 49
Sulfinpyrazone, 87
Sulfonamides, 86, 87

Talwin, 18, 144
Tandearil, 87
Terminal illness
  and drug therapy, 154, 203
Tetracyclines, 83, 84, 90, 114, 122, 135
Thioridazine, 16, 58, 144
Thiothixene, 143, 144
Thorazine, 18, 20, 58, 144, 200
Thyroid hormones, 122
Tofranil, 18, 60, 90, 144
Tolbutamide, 87, 88, 89
Tranquilizers, 16, 17, 18, 19, 20, 46, 47, 49, 88, 116, 120, 122, 127, 153, 154, 183, 193, 194, 200, 205, 206-207
  major, 16, 18, 20, 143, 144, 146, 147, 199
  minor, 16, 18, 47, 113, 143, 144, 146, 147
Transport of drugs (see Distribution of drugs)
Treatment of alcoholism, 35-36, 37, 38
Treatment for drug problems, 23, 25
Tricyclic antidepressants, 60-61, 89, 90, 143, 146
Trifluoperazine, 58, 144
Trilaphon, 58
Tuinal, 19, 46, 50
Tylenol, 144

Undermedication, 198, 199, 214

Valium, 18, 19, 46, 47, 50, 59, 60, 144, 165
Visual impairment, 6, 58, 59, 61, 67, 120, 165

Vitamins, 97
Vivactil, 60
Volunteer programs
   prevention of drug misuse, 185-187

Warfarin, 87

Wine
   sociability effects of, 37, 153, 202-203
Women (*see* Older women)

Young's Rule, 164, 212

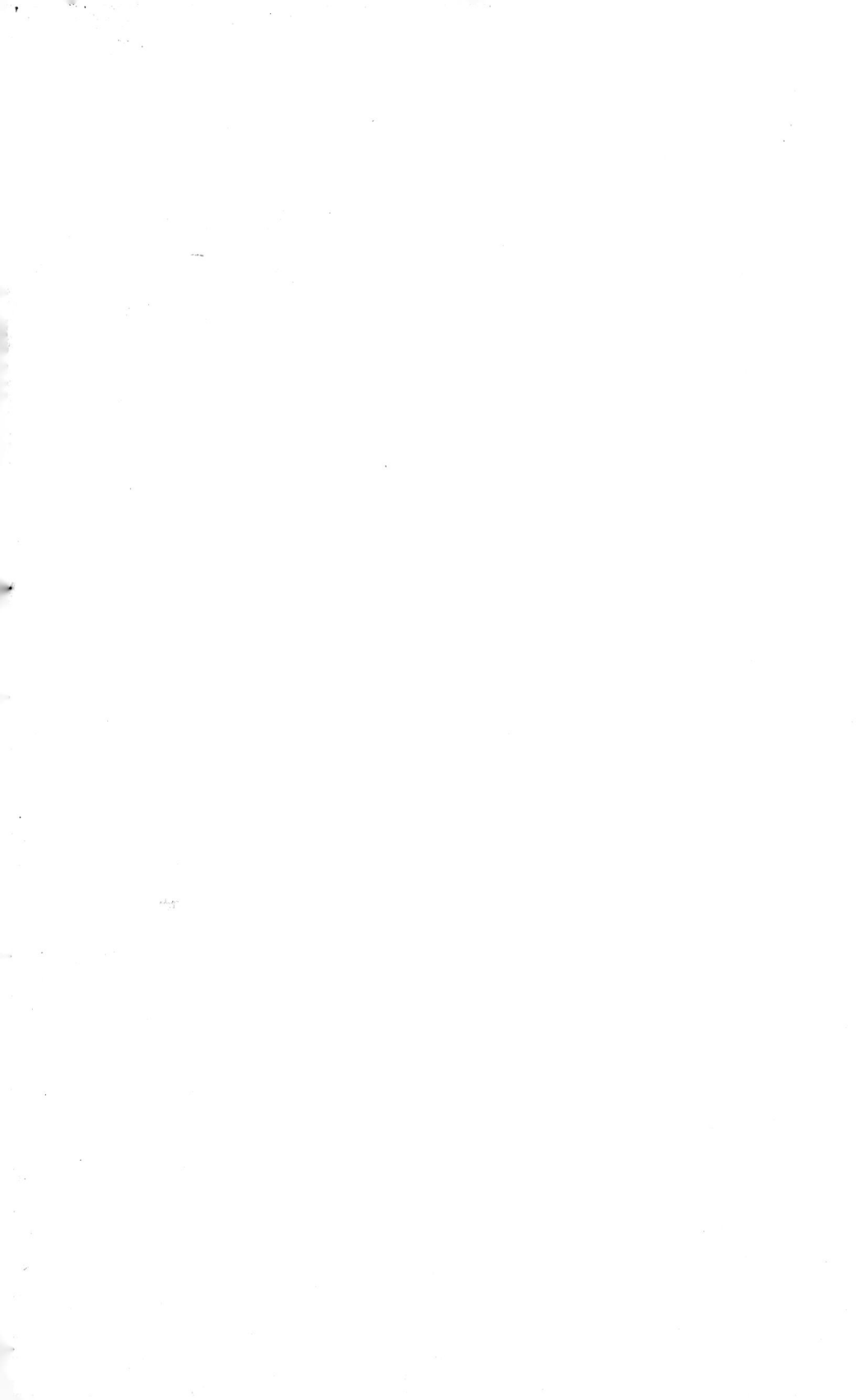